UNLOCKING
THE KILLER DISEASE
DIABETES

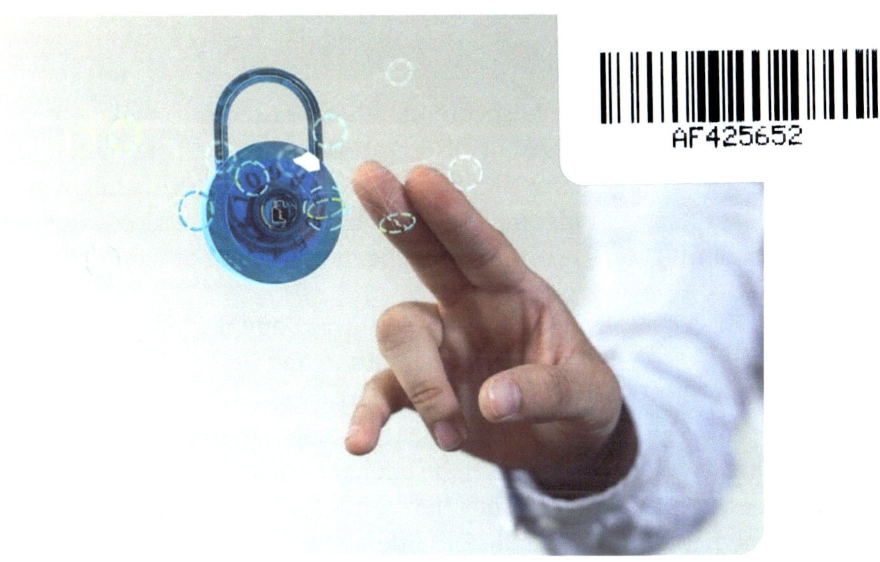

TALHA SARESHWALA

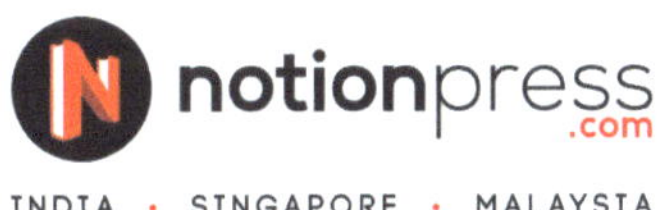

Unlocking the Killer Disease

Diabetes

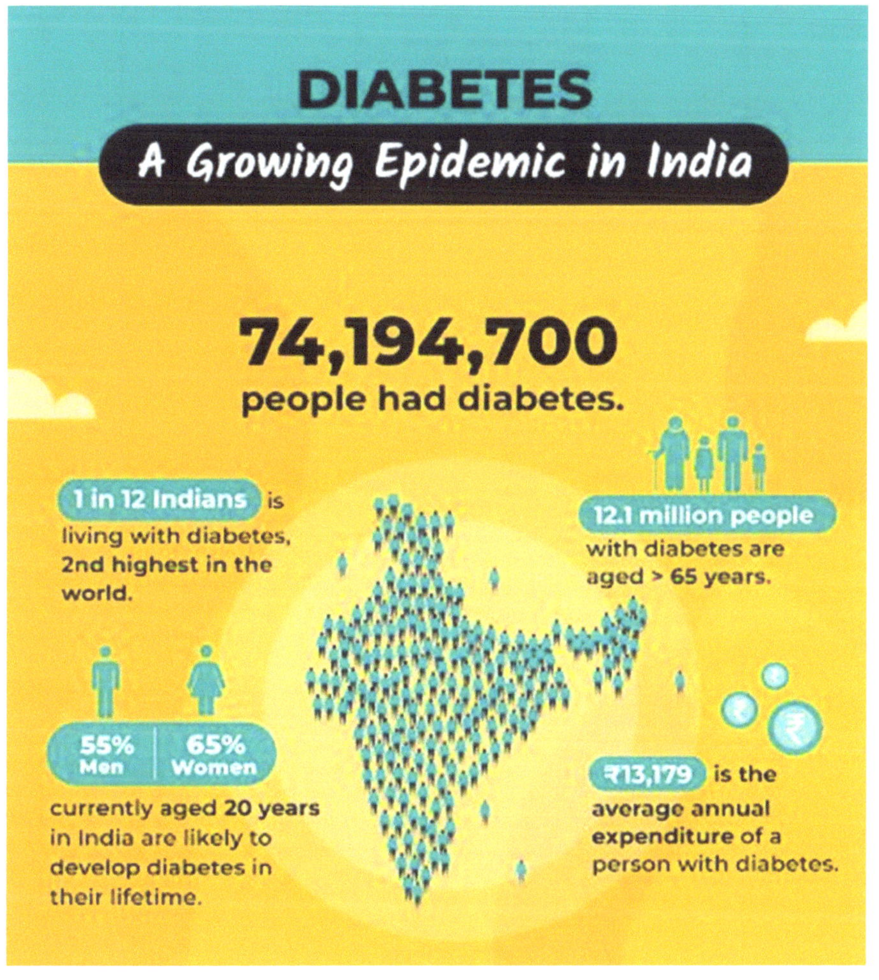

Disclaimer statements

1. The information in this Book is based on general information and does not substitute for an expert's advice. Author does not confirm this.

2. This Book is meant for information and Author's experience for sole purposes of Sharing only and must not be considered a substitute for advice provided by qualified medical professionals.

3. These articles in this Book are for generic purpose only and is no substitute to any doctor's advice.

Preface

It's been a year since I joined a reversal program for diabetes. This journey full of excitement, experiences, ups and down and most importantly a learning, process for me.

That is why, I thought of sharing my experiences as a Diabetic patient in this reversal journey through this book. UNLOCKING-The Killer Disease.

A Growing epidemic in India. 1 in 12 Indians is living with Diabetes, 2nd highest in the World. 12.1 million people with diabetes are aged more than 65 years. 55% Men and 65% Women currently aged 20 years in India are likely to develop diabetes in their lifetime. Rs 13,179 is the average annual expenditure of a person with diabetes

This book a non-fiction will be a riveting take on the world of Diabetes. Besides informative reading, it would also be a guide for Diabetic and Non Diabetics who wish to live a healthy and energetic lifestyle and make a difference in their living. It would offer its readers ideas and suggestions to take baby steps in Prevention and Cure, and to stay determined and focused to maintain a healthy Life.

A book that can act as a source of basic information for young and old Diabetes patients, while ensuring them that Discipline and change in Lifestyle through a strong willpower do pay in managing Diabetes when followed in true spirit and action. The book would also throw light on many crucial Diet and impact of Food, & Physical Exercise aspects so that it becomes useful in all senses.

1. Introduction- Unlocking the Diabetes

2. Empowering Your Health- As Simple as ABCD.......to keep Diabetes at Bay

3. Governing Blood Sugar

4. Diet- A Key To Your WellBeing

5. The Impact Of Food On Health and Well Being

6. Physical Activity- A key to Healthy Lifestyle

7. The Two Subordinates of Diabetes- Cholesterol & Obesity

8. Misconception About Diabetes- Know the Facts

Appendix

- Basic Diabetic Diet Regime

- Few Common Sense Health Tips

- Basic Suggestions for Healthy Life

I'm really excited to share my Book with esteemed Doctors and people in Medical fraternity and Diabetic Patients and all my well-wishers who helped make this book a reality. With all humility, I wish that all my readers contribute their feedback and opinion after reading the book. Your thoughts as a small note sharing your opinions on the subject would be a big plus.

The aim is to create a bank of diverse inputs, from the Medical fraternity which further enhances the subject's relevance.

I am sure your contribution/ feedback would help me in writing more books and to share my knowledge which becomes more interesting for readers to take advantage.

I would consider my endeavour worth all its efforts if it helps the Diabetic community or just a few and inspires them to follow disciplined lifestyle practices and make our country Diabetic free

Credits

I am eternally grateful to my **Late Father Mohd Yunus Sareshwala** for inspiring me and inculcating the habit of sharing and caring. **My Mother** for her never ending Duas (Prayer) and her blessings. Special thanks to **My Wife** and **2 daughters** for their relentless support and encouragement throughout the writing process. And not to forget to thank **Almighty Allah** as I couldn't have done anything without him. **Alhumdullilah Totally Grateful to him.**

This support gave me a thought of sharing my experience and knowledge as a Diabetic Patient through this Book **UNLOCKING - THE KILLER DISEASE.**

I am also extremly thankful to couple of Doctors who spared their valuable time in reading my manuscript and gave their very Honest and insightful views about my book. Their views have been printed as a testimonial and my personal satisfaction.

I have taken an Unusual approach in writing this book, in which information has been sourced and compiled from Internet, social media, attending various conferences, and webinars along with my thoughts, ideas, experiences and writing abilities.

RESEARCH & EDITORIAL:

Talha Sareshwala

PHOTOGRAPHS & GRAPHICS:

Free images from various Internet sites like @health-fuel, Shreya Shah; Google

CONTENT COMPILATION & EDIT:

- Dr V. Mohan Head of MDRF-Hinduja Foundation. Chairman and Cheif Diabetology, Diabetes specialities Centre
- Senior Dietician Care Hospitals Hyderabad
- Purnima Varghese Expert Diabetes Care and Management
- Neelanjana Singh, Nutrition and Wellness consultant
- The Indian Council of Medical Research (ICMR)
- Sumaiyya Khan (Welness Coach) Breathe Well Being (BWB) A Diabetes Reversal Program

BOOK LAYOUT AND DESIGN:

Notion Press

PRINTED AND PUBLISHED FOR:

PUBLISHER

TVS Partners

PRINTED AT

Notion Press

Dr. Iftekhar Sareshwala, MD (USA)
4000 Canyon Crest Rd,
San Ramon, CA 94582

Iftekhars2002@gmail.com

I have known Talha since childhood, and just like his dad Mr. Younus Sareshwala, (my uncle) Talha has always been a very detail oriented, well read person, knowledgeable and always curious about recent developments: specially in the medical field. Although a non-medico by profession, his hunger for medical knowledge over the years has been tremendous.

His recent book, "The Unlocking of killer disease Diabetes" is a very well written book with minimal medical jargon, easy to understand and thorough. As a medical professional in Internal Medicine and specializing in diabetes management myself, I found this book extremely informative, evidence based with easy to understand diagrams and charts.

Talha has put in a lot of effort collecting data from various medical journals and research papers and has displayed this in an immaculate manner. The chapter on diet and nutrition is very well written keeping the Indian dietary culture in mind. Also, the chapter on Myths and Misconception about diabetes would be an eye opener for the common man.

All in all, this book is a must read for the general public who wishes to understand and take control of this misunderstood and confusing disease.

I strongly recommend this book and feel that this is going to revolutionize the misconceptions about this extremely common, yet manageable disease.

Best Regards,

Iftekhar Sareshwala, MD (Internal Medicine)

Dr. Sonal Dalal (MDS)
Periodontal Surgeon
Certified Health and Wellness Coach

Heartiest congratulations for writing a remarkable book " The Unlocking Of Killer Diabetes "

As a healthcare professional and wellness coach I wanted to express my deepest appreciation for your insights into combating diabetes with sustainable lifestyle and holistic practices. It provides valuable strategies that I believe will significantly benefit many individuals striving to manage their health more. I look forward   to seeing the positive impact of your book on the health and wellness of community!

Dr Sonal Dalal
24thJune '24

Dr. Jayesh Raval (M.S., F.I.C.S.)
Cancer Surgeon
Specialised at Tata Memorial Hospital - Mumbai

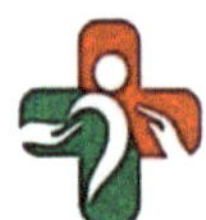

I just finished reading this very insightful and fascinating book – "The Unlocking of Killer Disease Diabetes". It is not only evidence based but also has a holistic approach to diabetes. It is written in simple language that can be understood by everyone. Glad to see you writing such an informative book on such a common yet not understood disease.

Bharati Hospital
Station Road, Patan - 384265
(H) 231309, 221168
drjayeshraval@yahoo.co.in | drravaljayesh@gmail.com

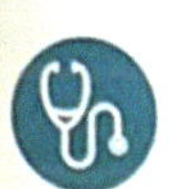

DEPARTMENT OF INTERNAL MEDICINE

Dr. Navneet Shah
MD (Medicine)
Sr. Diabetologist, Endocrinologist & Physician
Reg. No: G-8162, G-1301

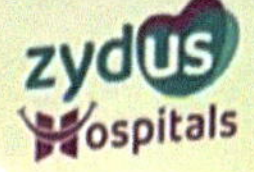

Date : 7/8/24

I had the opportunity to read the book written by Mr. Talha Sareshwala — "The unlocking of Killer of Disease Diabetes"

This book is very well written with excellant scientific content. This can be read and can be understood by common people.

It has lot of emphasis on Diet and its role in the management in the Diabetes mellitus Type 2.

In fact it has been written by the person who himself has undergone the agony of the disease and experienced the problem of its complications.

I strongly recommend to publish it for the larger interest of people suffering from Diabetes mellitus Type 2.

(Dr Navneet Shah)

Zydus Hospitals & Healthcare Research Pvt. Ltd.

Registered Office: Plot No. 232, Zydus Hospital Road, Thaltej, Ahmedabad- 380054, Gujarat, India | CIN U2433GJ2008PLC054191

For Appointment: +91 79 66190201   Emergency: +91 78744 12345   www.zydushospitals.com

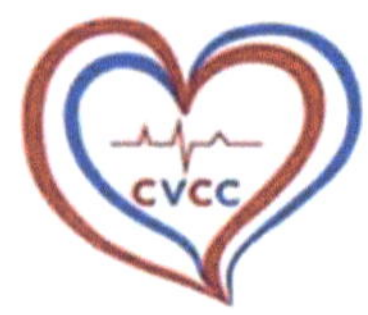

Hiren Patel, M.D., F.A.C.C.
Cardiology & Vascular Care Center
3115 Harbor Blvd, Port Charlotte, FL 33952
Phone: (941) 258-3635
Fax: (941) 258-3630

Talha, my childhood friend who I have known since our high school days, has always been a very detail oriented, well-read, and knowledgeable person.

His recent book, "The Unlocking of Killer Disease Diabetes" is a book that is thorough and makes it easy for a layman to understand what diabetes is. As a Cardiologist, I found this book extremely informative, written with a holistic approach and in an evidence based manner.

I highly recommend this book for the general public to understand and take control of this misunderstood and extremely common, yet manageable disease.

- Dr. Hiren Patel

Content

Chapter 1

INTRODUCTION - Unlocking The diabetes Code

Illness and disease can be heart breaking, difficult and test your faith. May Almighty cure all those suffering with visible and invisible illnesses.

–Ameen.

May Almighty grant a cure to all those who are unwell and in need of his healing. Ameen.

When we feel sick and are suffering from any pain, we remember how fragile we are and turn to our Creator. Almighty's Mercy is such that when in this state, you are shedding sins. Anything afflicting your body is helping you spiritually. True understanding is that Almighty is responsible for everything happening all the time, and that His plan is from divine wisdom. You may feel sick and terrible for a few days or weeks but once healed, you will be free of some of the sins of the past. Alhamdulillah (Gratitude) for the blessings of our Lord!

My personal beleif of taking a holistic approach to health helps better manage not only the symptoms that arise, but also the root causes. These often include repetitive daily motion, inactivity, and overwork. Plus, it helps manage the emotional burden that comes with chronic pain.

Holistic health is an approach to wellness that simultaneously addresses the physical, mental, emotional, social, and spiritual components of health. As a field of practice, holistic medicine draws from many disciplines, religions, and cultures to heal people, communities, and even the environment, approach to wellness can not only help boost productivity, mental clarity, physical health but also resilience to face challenges of daily life headstrong.

May Almighty God heal the sick and the unwell including those in hospital, those suffering from various illness and stress. May Almighty make it easy for us all. Always have hope and remain hopeful in God's mercy.... Ameen!

Here I take the liberty as an example from Holy Quran and Hadiths about holistic approach to illness.

Beautiful Hadith is about the Cure of an Illness.

Narrated Abu Hurairah (RA): The Prophet (SAW) said, "There is no disease that Allah has created, except that He also has created its treatment." (Sahih Bukhari Book 71 Hadith 582)

Surah Al-Fateh (A Quranic Chapter) is known as the opening of the Quran. It is also known as Surah us Shifa, the healing chapter.

We all fall ill at some time and it can seem as though the world's falling apart when we're low, but remember Allah is the One who created the illness and the cure. When you are sick, your Duas are more precious so use them. When you are afflicted with something, the reward is greater so know that you are gaining blessings for every second of your sickness. Even the diseases of the heart have a treatment in remembrance of Allah, so if spiritual illnesses can be cured so can physical ones. If you are healthy, say Alhamdulillah Gratitude to God and pray for all those who are unwell. Every religion encourages us to stay healthy and look after our bodies.

The last few years coupled with the recent pandemic have been instrumental in accelerating the urgency **for mental health awareness** and has led to significant digital and technological innovations addressing the service delivery gaps.

"Depression, anxiety and panic attacks are not signs of weakness. They are sign of illness." Mental health is not a stigma: But to not have your suffering recognized and diagnosed is an almost unbearable form of violence."

Depression can be dangerous. Bit by bit, day by day it can slowly grow before it overwhelms & controls you. Be positive in every outlook of your life. If you feel life isn't as planned, be assured that you are exactly where Allah wants you to be. And He is the best of planners. Mental Health has largely remained in the fringes in India, due to its deep-rooted stigma, taboo, and myths. This has resulted in limited access to mental health services and shortage of such specialists. Anxiety attacks & depression can happen to any of us. It's a sad reality; And also, who like me continue to fight diabetes or even have diabetes themselves, and dreadful disease of CANCER; support them and help them in disciplined life style, workouts, and healthy diet. So be one and unite to fight these progressive diseases thus, it's essential to reach out to each other.

Islam encourages believers to help each other through whatever means possible "They will be asked, What's wrong with you? Why do you not help each other? ("**Quran 37:25**).

Certainly, in these most difficult moments of life you realize who are true friends or people who really appreciate you. I have decided to ponder on these diseases just to make people aware of the horrific by-products of diabetes. The disease ruins your cardiovascular and renal systems.... And the drugs, that are prescribed, may encourage the onset of dementia. Diabetes is very invasive and destructive to our body, even after treatment, and medications your body is still struggling with yourself trying to regulate the spiking/dropping of blood sugar levels all the time. It's a very long process.

Type 2 diabetes is one of the world's biggest health threats and India is the capital of it. **The study by The Indian Council of Medical Research (ICMR)** 1 in 12 Indians are suffering from this lifestyle disorder in India, and another 136 million are prediabetic. In type 2 diabetes, a person is either unable to produce enough insulin for energy or it doesn't use the insulin produced for energy. The symptoms include increased thirst, frequent urination, hunger, fatigue and blurred vision. In some cases, there may be no symptoms. Managing your diet, exercise, medication and insulin therapy are the treatments available for it. Though it is a chronic progressive disease, it is reversible.

Similarly, after chemotherapy treatment, it's true that it takes years to feel alive... with the side effects of the chemotherapy and radiation, you will never be back to 100% because of the weakened immune system. Sure, in the most difficult moments of life you realize who your real friends are or the people who really appreciate you. Cancer is a very invasive and destructive enemy of our bodies. After the end of the treatment, the body remains devastated. Recovery from the damage caused by the treatment of the disease is a very long process.

Truly it's imperative for us to honour a family member or a friend who died of cancer, or still fighting cancer, how many times have we heard others say: "if you need anything, don't hesitate to call me, I'll be there to help you" and show your support to the family / friend who can wrestle.

I really and truly feel the need to encourage employers/leaders/managers to think about introducing a prayer/meditation room to be used by all their employees in the interest of diversity and mental health and well-being. It'll enhance work output and potentially improve employee morale and retention too. Meditation can produce a deep state of **relaxation** and a tranquil mind. During meditation, you focus your attention and eliminate the stream of jumbled thoughts that may be crowding your mind and causing stress. This process may result in enhanced physical and emotional well-being.

Prevention is Better than Cure

What is your opinion on "Prevention is better than Cure."

Here prevention is our journey which we take for the reversal and Cure is the Medicines which we take.

Believe me looking after your body and health is a religious imperative. Be sure to watch what you eat, exercise however you can, and take care of the body Almighty God gave you so that you are fit and healthy for family, for worship and for yourself.

Diet and Nutrition play a big part in maintaining the best possible health, so does a lifestyle incorporating exercise. Create a self-belief and lay emphasis on a simple diet combined with physical exercise as advised by your respective coaches.

"Protection of life and health is second in merit after preservation of one's religion.

Protecting Oneself from Injury, Danger, Sickness, Harm and Accidents is a Religious Obligation.

Seeking Treatment and Medication for Health is a Religious Imperative.

"God is the Creator of both sickness and medicine. He has stipulated a cure for every sickness therefore seek out treatment [for good health and well-being]!"

My Journey My Experience of Reversal Diabetes

Now, let me share a little story from my own journey. I was in a similar boat with my HbA1c Levels creeping up. I was already on medication, but I wanted to try some natural methods too. So, I got an opportunity to attend a webinar on Diabetes Reversal Programme, sounded interesting and attractive to give a try…..Diabetes Reversal is a program claiming to address the root cause of diabetes by targeting fat cells that disrupt insulin production. It promotes weight loss, dietary adjustments, and specific meal timings with Portion Control to regulate blood sugar levels. However, its effectiveness and safety may vary for individuals. Before starting any new diabetes management program, it's crucial to consult with healthcare professionals to ensure it aligns with your overall treatment plan.

And I think age has nothing to do with diabetes. It is only your mindset which decides whether you are going to fight back or not. I personally took it as a challenge, Joined the programme and started making small changes to my diet, now I'm able to control my cravings by eating something healthy. I see and meet many people at restaurants as well, where they eat anything of their choice but I still stick to my diet which is 1 or 2 roti, 1 sabzi, 1 dal and 1 bowl of salad.

So this is the combination that I followed from the beginning. I rarely crossed 900 to 950 calories per day, because as per me that's not something that I'm really keeping a track of, the lower the calories the better for me, it can be different for you. If you have any concerns regarding your diet, you can ask your nutrionalist and customise it as per your comfort and requirements.

I also used to check my sugars after 2 hours of it, but with god's grace, it has never increased.

Plus whenever you're having food, make sure that you avoid oil as much as possible, use very little maybe 1 or 2 teaspoon max to prepare your food. I am not a rice eater, so this was my primary diet.

I gave up all of sugar also completely kicked my sugar tooth, and all simple carbohydrates, completely eliminating processed foods, to this day, I no longer like things that are very sweet, and I am able to have a small sweet treat without wanting to eat every sugary thing I can get my hands on. It was a challenging month in which I discovered a lot of foods I'd never known. I ate a lot of nuts and lean meat, but also came to appreciate things like Bitter Gourd, Brussels sprouts and cauliflower, and lot of leafy vegetables both of which I love now. swapping out snacks for healthier options, and adding more veggies to my meals. Plus whenever I am having food, I make sure that I avoid oil as much as possible, use very little maybe 1 or 2 teaspoon max, FOR STARTERS dry stuffs, I ALWAYS PREFER STUFF MADE IN Air Fryer.

Followed a strict diet regime curated by my nutritionalist....so this was my primary diet.

- **Early morning 5 or 6 am** - Any drink of your choice as per the diet plan - I used to drink only Methi Dana Water, and Dalchini water to detox my body, also took Kalonji Oil (Black Seed) mix in Black Tea........ you can drink what works for you.

- **Breakfast 7 30 am** - Any combination of breakfast as per your diet plan - I have 1 Jau Roti, any form of egg 1 glass of Cucumber Smoothie & 1 bowl of salad. On other days I used to have 2 to 3 Chilas, 1 bowl of Chutney, 1 glass of Cucumber Smoothie & 1 bowl of salad.

- **Lunch 1 30 pm** - Any combination of lunch as per your diet plan - I have 2 Jau Roti, 1 sabzi,(Leafy vrgetables) 1 dal or Chicken Curry once or twice in a week & 1 bowl of salad. On other days I used to have 2 to 3 Chilas, 1 bowl of Chutney, 1 dal & 1 bowl of salad.

- **Evening Snack 4 or 5 pm** - Combination of some seeds and nuts - I have 1 teaspoon of seeds given to me as per my diet like Pumkin Seeds Sunflower Seeds Flax Seeds and on other days I used to have 7-9 soaked almonds after peeling them and 1 whole walnut. On some more other days I used to have 1 bowl or makhane or roasted chana or Peanuts.

- **Dinner 7 or 7 30 pm**- Any combination of dinner as per your diet plan - I have 2 Jau Roti, 1 sabzi, 1 dal & 1 bowl of salad. On other days I used to have 2 to 3 Chilas, 1 bowl of Chutney, 1 dal & 1 bowl of salad.

I also committed to taking a daily walk, light physical excersise rain or shine. It wasn't easy at first, but gradually I started to notice a difference. I'm 5'7" and I was 68 Kgs when I started and 60 at the end of the month, and feel as physically youthful as I did when I was in my late 30's or early 40's. My energy levels improved, and sure enough, when I went for my next check-up, my HbA1c had dropped. It was such a great feeling knowing that I was taking control of my health in a positive way. So hang in there, stay consistent, and you'll see results before you know it! I've learned a lot more about nutrition and healthy eating since then, but it was a formative month in both physiologically shifting my body's response to no sugar, and strict diet plan and psychologically proving to myself that I can stick to a strict eating plan. Both of these things have enabled me to stick with more balanced, healthier eating since the month of my reversal programme.

I want to say that taking charge of my health like this was a big deal. It's awesome that I started looking for ways to bring down my HbA1c levels.

Alright, so if you have got a high HbA1c level and you're already on tablets. That's a good start because medication can definitely help manage blood sugar levels. But, do try about adding some natural approaches into the mix, just like what I did. One thing I've found super helpful was tweaking my diet, try to focus on foods that are low on the glycemic index. Think veggies, lean proteins, and healthy fats. Also, regular exercise can work wonders. It doesn't have to be anything crazy - even just a daily walk can make a big difference. And don't underestimate the power of stress management techniques like meditation or yoga. Stress can wreak havoc on blood sugar levels, so finding ways to chill out can really help. Remember, it's all about finding what works best for you and sticking with it. You've got this!

What is Diabetes

In simple words, Diabetes is a condition where the body does not properly process food for use as energy. Most of the food we eat is turned into glucose, or sugar, for our bodies to use for energy. The pancreas, an organ that lies near the stomach, makes a hormone called insulin to help glucose get into the cells of our bodies.

> A disease in which the body's ability to produce or respond to the hormone Insulin is impaired, resulting in abnormal

metabolism of carbohydrates leading to elevated levels of glucose in the blood and Urine.

A condition in which the body does not properly process food for use as energy. The food we eat is turned into glucose/sugar. Insulin helps push the glucose from the blood stream into the tissues and cells.

Elevated blood glucose is secondary to either decrease or absent Insulin OR because of a condition referred to as Insulin Resistance.

The most common types of diabetes are type 1, type 2, and gestational diabetes.

Type 1 diabetes

If you have type 1 diabetes your body does not make insulin. Your immune system attacks and destroys the cells in your pancreas that make insulin. Type 1 diabetes is usually diagnosed in children and young adults, although it can appear at any age. People with type 1 diabetes need to take insulin every day to stay alive.

Type 2 diabetes

If you have type 2 diabetes your body does not make or use insulin well. You can develop type 2 diabetes at any age, even during childhood. However, this type of diabetes occurs most often in middle-aged and older people. Type 2 is the most common type of diabetes.

Gestational diabetes

Gestational diabetes develops in some women when they are pregnant. Most of the time, this type of diabetes goes away after the baby is born. However, if you've had gestational diabetes, you have a greater chance of developing type 2 diabetes later in life.

Diabetes care is not rocket science.

Look at your glycosylated hemoglobin (A1C). Is it under 7?

Look at your morning fasting blood sugars. Are they typically below 120?

Do you understand how to eat a diabetic diet?

It might be a good idea to see an endocrinologist if:

1   You are a type 2 diabetic.

2   You are a MODY.

3   You don't have a good understanding of how to deal with your illness and you never got an opportunity to get any education.

4   You are not at goal A1C after repeated efforts to "get there."

Why not source some authentic information?" This is not to imply that you are ignorant, but a nice, easy, simple source of knowledge which has a lot of information and facts may be just the right thing for you. Also, go to the diabetic classes. Most hospitals have them. Most doctors don't refer "run of the mill" diabetes. More commonly, they will refer patients who are difficult to treat or who need more intensive education.

The exact cause of diabetes is unknown, but researchers believe that it is a combination of genetics, lifestyle, and environmental factors that can contribute to its onset. Genetics plays a role in both type 1 and type 2 diabetes. Researchers have identified certain genes that may make some individuals more likely to develop diabetes. In addition, lifestyle and environmental factors, such as diet, physical activity, and exposure to certain toxins, may increase an individual's risk of developing diabetes.

The prevalence of diabetes is increasing globally and is a major public health concern. It is estimated that over 420 million people around the world are living with diabetes, and this number is projected to increase to over 642 million by 2040. Diabetes is a leading cause of death and disability, and can result in serious health complications, including heart disease, stroke, kidney failure, also individuals with Type 2 diabetes are at a higher risk of developing other serious health conditions, such as vision loss and amputations, and nerve damage.

The best way to prevent or delay the onset of diabetes is to maintain a healthy lifestyle. This includes eating a balanced diet, exercising regularly, and avoiding smoking and excessive alcohol consumption. In addition, people with a family history of diabetes should be screened regularly for high blood glucose levels. Early diagnosis and treatment can help reduce the risk of developing diabetes-related complications.

Over time, the body can become resistant to the effects of insulin, and the blood sugar levels can become dangerously high.

In addition, The best way to reduce the risk of complications from diabetes is to follow a healthy lifestyle, maintain healthy blood sugar levels, and work closely with your healthcare provider.

Certainly, in these most difficult moments of life you realize who are true friends or people who really appreciate you. I have decided to ponder on these diseases just to make people aware of the horrific by-products of diabetes. The disease ruins your cardiovascular and renal systems.... And the drugs, that are prescribed, may encourage the onset of dementia. Diabetes is very invasive and destructive to our body, even after treatment, and medications your body is still struggling with yourself trying to regulate the spiking/dropping of blood sugar levels all the time. It's a very long process.

Well being

The demanding nature of TODAY'S profession AND Life STYLE is a stark reminder that chronic stress can silently deteriorate our well-being and highlights the urgent need for stress management techniques.

Warranty Expires at 40:

It's time to emphasizes the importance of proactive health measures, particularly after age 40. Our bodies, much like an engine, come with a limited warranty. Beyond this threshold, we must invest extra effort in self-care and regular health check-ups to maintain our overall well-being and prevent potential heart-related issues.

Sleep and Diet-Pillars of Overall Health :

The significance of maintaining a healthy lifestyle through two essential pillars:

Quality sleep.

A balanced diet.

Prioritizing sufficient sleep and nourishing our bodies with wholesome food can significantly reduce the risk of heart-related complications.

Insulin resistance(IR)

Insulin resistance is when, your cells stop responding properly to insulin resulting in high blood sugar levels.

IR is a very common contributor to Type2 Diabetes & cardiovascular disease.

What is Insulin?

Insulin is a hormone produced by beta cells of the pancreas.

The name insulin comes from the Latin ''insula'' for "island" from the cells that produce the hormone in the pancreas.

What does insulin do?

After we eat food & it's digested, it will be converted into sugar, which will be used as energy.

Insulin is a key that unlocks the door of our cell wall so sugar can enter, Once insulin (unlocks) the cell wall, sugar can move into the cells for energy.

THE ROLE OF INSULIN IN THE BODY

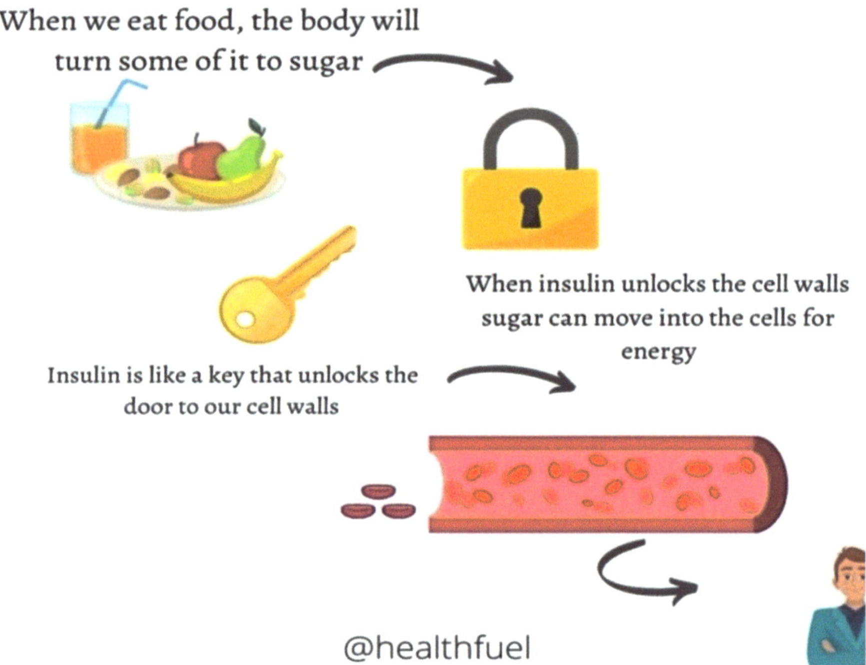

Insulin resistance

In case of insulin resistance, the cell receptors(locks) are jammed/ there is not enough insulin(keys), leaving the glucose locked out and swimming in the blood streams. This causes high blood sugar.

The problem is defective cell receptors or not enough insulin.

So, Insulin resistance is when cells in your muscles, fat, and liver don't respond well to insulin and can't use glucose from your blood for energy.

INSULIN RESISTANCE

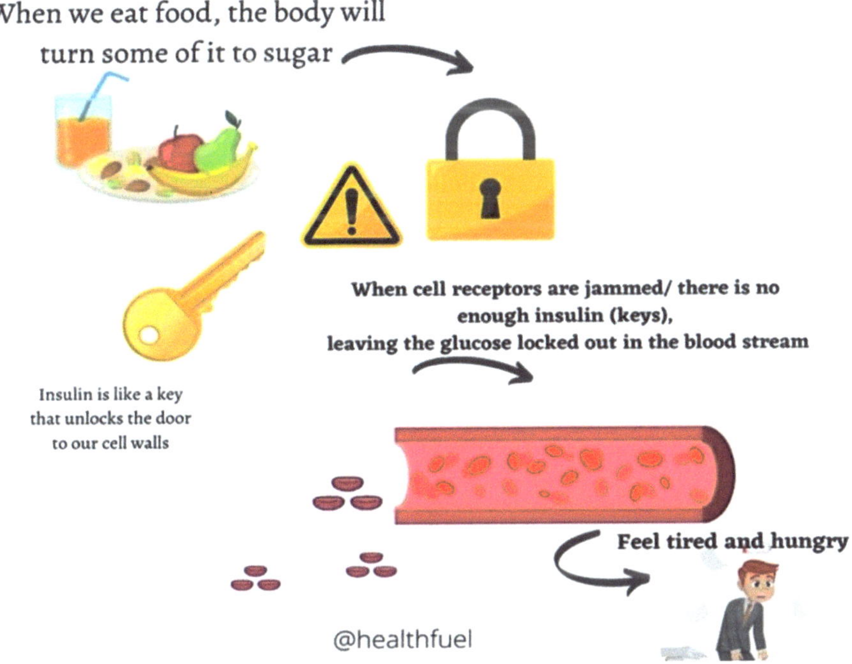

To make up for it, your pancreas makes more insulin. Over time, your blood sugar levels go up and an overproduction of insulin.

Risk Factors

Yes, diet and weight are 2 important factors. But it's important to note that there are many other factors associated to IR.

- Family history of Diabetes.

- Physical inactivity.

- Hormonal imbalance (thyroid or PCOS).

- Low HDL(Good cholesterol).

- Stress

- Poor Sleep

RISK FACTORS AND INSULIN RESISTANCE

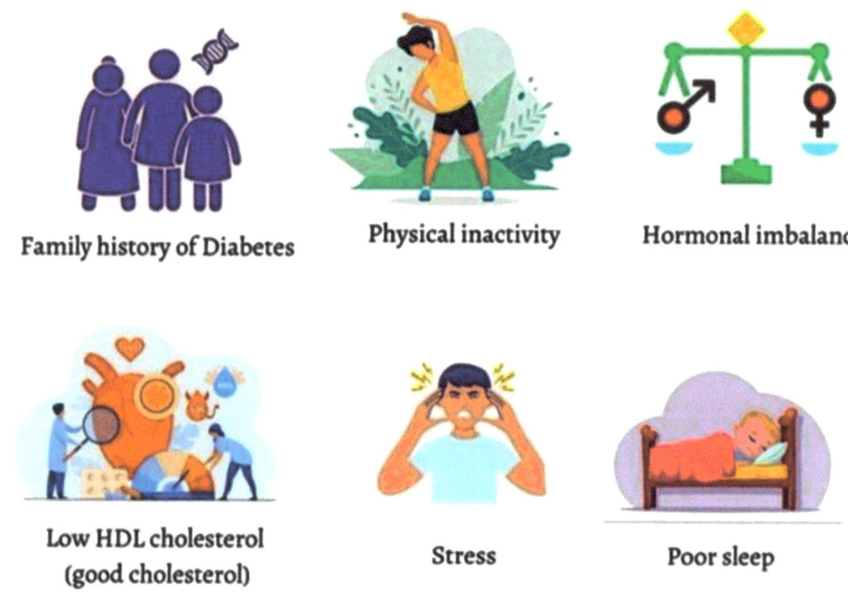

@healthfuel

How do you find out if you're insulin resistant?

No one test will tell you, but high blood sugar levels, high triglycerides, high LDL cholesterol, & low HDL cholesterol, may determine you have IR.

You can test for fasting insulin, fasting blood glucose, HBA1c& a lipid profile.

Developing IR is a gradual progression that builds up over the course of many years before it manifests and you are diagnosed with prediabetes or type2 diabetes.

Improving Insulin sensitivity can help prevent more chronic conditions but also promote highest state of health.

Dietary & lifestyle guidelines to manage insulin resistance

If you have IR, you want to become the opposite—more insulin sensitive (cells are more effective at absorbing blood sugar so less insulin is needed).

Weight management: weight loss can also cut down on insulin resistance.

Excess weight, especially the abdominal fat, reduces insulin sensitivity weight loss is an effective way to increase insulin sensitivity.

Reduce Added Sugar Intake

Do a kitchen assessment to become aware of all of the hidden sources of sugar that are sneaking into your eating plan.

Avoid Drinking Liquid Sugar

Almost half of the added sugar comes from beverages like coffee with sugar — such as vanilla Latte & mochas, fruit drinks, soda,& other sweetened beverages.

Liquid sugar is absorbed in the body more rapidly than added sugar found in foods.

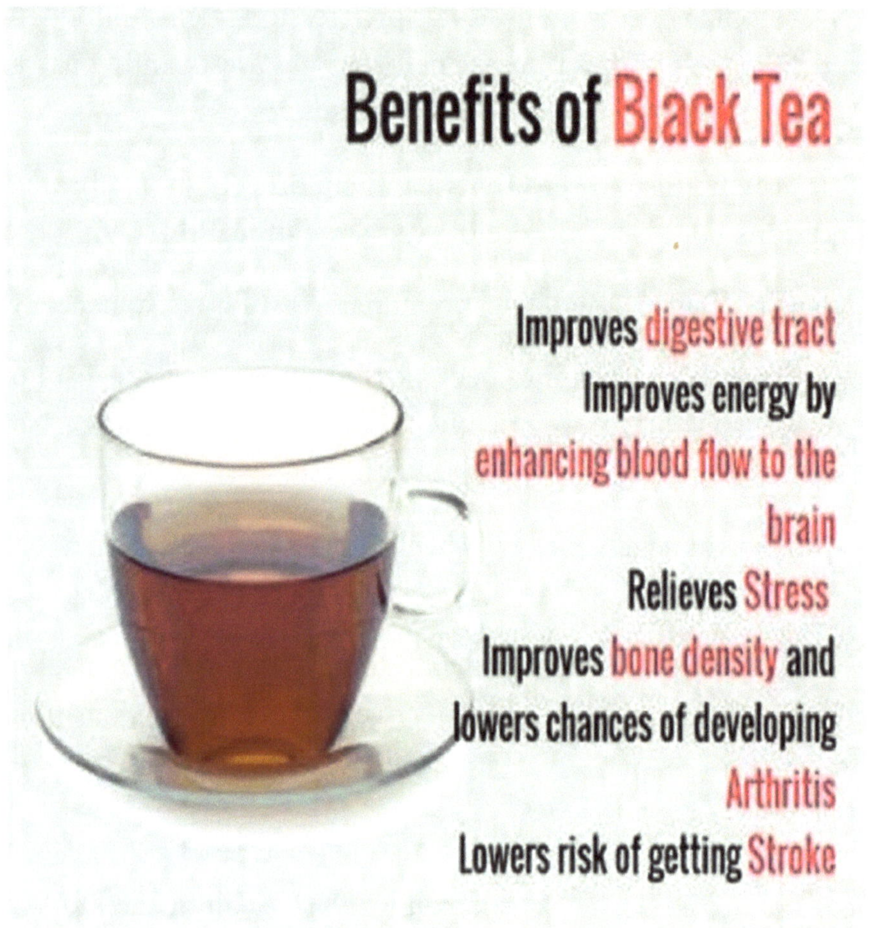

Carbohydrates

- Avoid eating carbohydrates alone, pair it with good quality protein & fat.

- Avoid refined flours and refined grains.

- Eating complex carbs, spreading your carb intake throughout the day, and choosing low-GI carbs are smart ways to increase insulin sensitivity.

- A diet that is Low carb, high protein, and good fats is recommended for managing insulin resistance.

- When you go low-carb, you also need to make sure that you balance it out with quality proteins and fats.

Eat more soluble fiber

Fiber can be divided into 2 categories, soluble&insoluble.

Insoluble fiber mostly acts as a bulking agent to help stool move through the bowels.

Soluble fiber is responsible for many of fiber's benefits,like lowering cholesterol&reducing appetite.

soluble fiber is found in nuts, seeds, non-starchy vegetables, low glycemic fruit and legumes.

Exercise

Physical activity makes you more sensitive to insulin, one reason why it's a cornerstone of IR management.

Exercise regularly, walk/take a stroll every 45min.

Cardiovascular exercise for 30-45 min(5-6 days/week.

Strength training 10-30min (3 days/week).

Sleep

Research shows that when you sleep, you repair your cells, regulate your satiety hormones and improve your insulin sensitivity.

Prioritise high quality sleep and 7-8 hours per night.

Prioritise Stress Reduction

Over time, chronic stress can keep blood sugar levels elevated. As a result, fat cells become less sensitive to insulin.

This increases the body's inclination to store fat and contributes to insulin resistance.

Conclusion

Insulin is an imp hormone that has many roles in the body.

IR may result in high blood sugar, which r thought to increase ur risk for diabetes&heart disease.

I have highlighted the dietary&lifestyle changes, along with regular exercise is the key in management of IR.

Pre-diabetes!!

As the name suggests, pre-diabetes is a stage just before diabetes.

Your body has started showing functional changes similar to diabetes but not high enough for it to be diagnosed as Diabetes.

There is a very high prevalence of pre-diabetes in India.

The scariest being teens who are not more than 15-16years of age are struggling with this just as much as older people.

Most people stay pre-diabetic for 5-10 years before getting diagnosed.

Are you at risk??

Our body is usually good at giving signs if there is an existing issue internally.

I'm sharing these signs/ risk factors/ Symptoms in the picture below.

If your score is more than 2 it calls for immediate attention!!

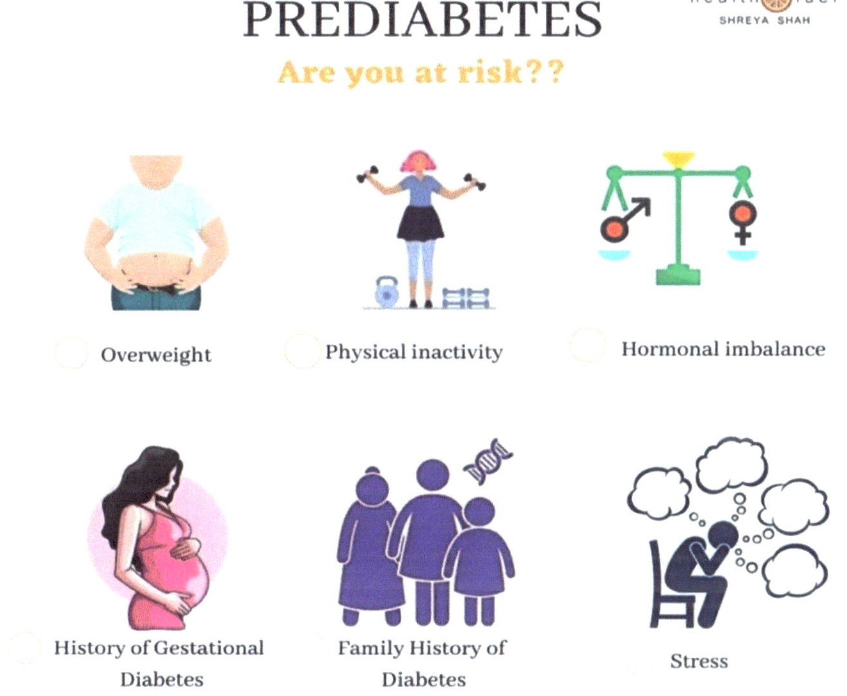

Now, that you know what pre-diabetes is,and the risk factors, the next step is to identify,if you're a pre-diabetic.

You can identify pre-diabetes with some basic blood investigation.

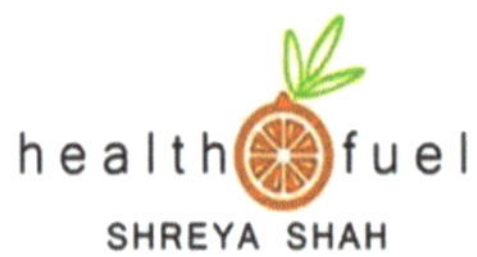

DIAGNOSTIC CRITERIA

Normal, Pre-diabetes, Diabetes

Sr.No.	PARAMETERS	NORMAL	PRE-DIABETES	DIABETES
1.	Fasting Plasma Blood glucose (mg/dl)	<100	100-125	≥126
2.	2hrs. Plasma blood glucose or OGTT (mg/dl) (75gm of glucose)	<140	IMPAIRED GLUCOSE TOLERANCE 140 - 199	≥200
3.	HbA1c (%)	<5.7	5.7-6.4	≥6.5

Typically, people with prediabetes do not show symptoms, are unaware that they have it& never have their blood sugar tested.

It is recommended to screen for most adults from age 30 & before that(even about 20 years)if one is overweight & has additional risk factors for prediabetes.

Can Prediabetes be prevented or avoided?

Prediabetes can be delayed &, in some cases, even prevented.

When people are overweight, losing weight and maintaining a healthy diet and exercise are the usual methods used to manage the condition.

Management of Pre-diabetes

So here are a few starter steps to prevent or reverse pre-diabetes.

These will obviously improve your diabetes, PCOS, weight, cholesterol issues, anxiety, and gut issues.

Healthy eating plan for prediabetes.

Full half of your plate with non-starchy veg - this will keep your overall carb intake low, high fibre will ensure you get host of phytonutrients.

Include Healthy fat

- Fat stabilizes blood sugars, this helps in keeping your insulin levels lower & hence less stress in the pancreas to produce insulin.

- By fat I mean the real, natural foods that happen to contain fat, not the processed food.

- Eg: nuts & seeds, avocado, fatty fish.

Protein

When you eat carb in combination with protein&healthy fat,it can take longer for ur body to convert the carbs into glucose,leading to lower post-meal blood sugar levels.

Protein reduces the calorie intake by providing satiety,which also helps in blood sugar control.

Low muscle mass is a contributor to insulin resistance.

Try to get protein in every meal for maximum benefit.

The best sources of proteins are dairy products like milk, curd, paneer as well as eggs, fish&poultry.

Avoid

  – processed foods

  – simple carbs like refined flour(maida), refined sugar

  – sugary drinks and fruit juices

  – High carbohydrate meal

Exercise

Exercise helps control weight, manage blood pressure,lower triglycerides, raise healthy HDL cholesterol,strengthen muscles,&improve ur general well-being.

Exercise lowers blood glucose levels & boosts your body's sensitivity to insulin, countering insulin resistance.

All forms of exercise—aerobic, resistance/doing both (combined training)—were equally good at lowering HbA1c values. The goal is to get at least 150 minutes per week of moderate-intensity activity.

One way to do this is to try to fit in at least 20-25 min of activity/day.

Manage your stress

Chronic stress can wreak havoc on health and well-being, stress hormones like cortisol can contribute to weight gain and elevated blood sugar.

Add stretching exercises, meditation or deep-breathing exercises to your daily routine.

Prioritize Sleep

Getting inadequate amounts of sleep can negatively impact blood sugar levels, short and long term.

Too little sleep puts stress on your body, causing it to release hormones, including cortisol.Cortisol increases insulin resistance & blood sugar levels.

Conclusion

Prediabetes if uncontrolled can open a Pandora's box full of diseases for you.

So, I strongly recommend getting yourself diagnosed and start these lifestyle changes, if you have more than 2 of the above mentioned risk factors.

Chapter 2

Empowering your Health: As simple as **ABCD…… to keep diabetes at bay**

Are you sitting for more than 10 hours, working or watching screen, and making no efforts to exercise or go for a walk? You could be raising your risk of diabetes, one of the fastest-growing diseases in the world that could be linked to your lifestyle choices. Coupled with unhealthy eating habits like low-fibre, high fat, and sugary diet, and modern-day stress, diabetes could strike even earlier than expected. Once diagnosed, diabetes Management is a life-long exercise as uncontrolled blood sugar levels can wreak havoc with both mental and physical health. As per WHO, about 422 million people have diabetes around the world and almost 1.5 million deaths are directly attributed to diabetes annually.

More people are at risk of diabetes than ever before due to their faulty lifestyle choices, and to prevent the disease, it would require conscious efforts every day. However, it's possible to avoid diabetes if you are walking regularly, eating a balanced diet with fibre, protein and other essential food groups, managing your stress levels, sleeping well and avoiding smoking and alcohol.

Dr. V. Mohan, Head of MDRF-Hinduja Foundation T1D program and also Chairman & Chief of Diabetology, Dr. Mohan's Diabetes Specialities Centre & President, Madras Diabetes Research Foundation, Chennai, India in an interview with HT talks extensively about lifestyle changes that can help us keep diabetes at bay.

Why do Blood sugar tend to increase even when you have not consume any food.

As a Doctor of Medicine, I can provide you with some insights into why your blood sugar may rise when you don't eat. The regulation of blood sugar levels is a complex process involving various hormones and organs in the body, primarily the pancreas and the liver.

When you don't eat for an extended period, your body still needs a constant supply of glucose (sugar) for energy. Glucose is the primary source of energy for cells, especially for the brain. In a well-regulated system, the body maintains blood sugar levels within a narrow range through the actions of insulin and other hormones.

Here are a few reasons why your blood sugar may increase when you don't eat:

1. **Glycogen Breakdown:** Your body stores glucose in the form of glycogen in the liver and muscles. When you don't eat, especially for an extended period, your body starts breaking down glycogen into glucose to maintain blood sugar levels.

2. **Gluconeogenesis:** In the absence of dietary carbohydrates, your body can produce glucose from non-carbohydrate sources, such as amino acids (building blocks of proteins) and glycerol (from fats). This process is known as gluconeogenesis.

3. **Hormonal Response:** Hormones play a crucial role in regulating blood sugar levels. When you don't eat, insulin levels decrease, and other hormones like glucagon and cortisol increase. These hormones work to raise blood sugar by promoting the release of glucose from the liver and inhibiting glucose uptake by cells.

4. **Stress Response:** Stress, whether physical or emotional, can lead to an increase in blood sugar levels. The body perceives fasting as a stressor, leading to the release of stress hormones that elevate blood sugar.

It's important to note that individual responses to fasting can vary, and factors such as overall health, insulin sensitivity, and pre-existing medical conditions can influence how your body manages blood sugar levels during periods of not eating.

If you're experiencing persistent or extreme fluctuations in blood sugar levels, it's crucial to consult with a healthcare professional. They can conduct specific tests, evaluate your medical history, and provide personalised advice on managing blood sugar levels to ensure your overall health and well-being.

Lifestyle changes for diabetes

Diabetes mellitus is a disorder that is known for disrupting the way your body uses glucose. It also causes other problems with the way your body stores and processes other forms of energy, including fat. Can be due to Insulin resistance and relative or absolute insulin deficiency. Diabetes is a growing global health concern that affects millions of people worldwide. While there is no sure-fire way to guarantee you won't develop diabetes, there are proven strategies that can significantly reduce your risk. Lifestyle changes play a pivotal role in diabetes prevention.

People with diabetes require regular monitoring and ongoing treatment to maintain goal blood sugar levels. Treatment includes lifestyle adjustments, self-care measures, and medications.

1. Eat balanced diet

What you are eating can greatly affect your chances of getting diabetes. While high-carb and high-sugar diet with little or no fibre can put you at increased risk of getting the metabolic disorder, a balanced diet with the right nutrients can help you in shedding kilos, nourishing your body and balancing your blood sugar levels. It is important to include a lot of fibre-rich foods in your diet like whole grains, fruits, vegetables, and legumes. Fibre helps control blood sugar and promotes a feeling of fullness.

If you have a sweet tooth, you should reconsider the sources from where you are satiating your cravings as refined sugars and simple carbohydrates can play havoc with your blood sugar levels. It is important to eliminate sugary snacks, sodas, and processed foods from your diet and go for complex carbohydrates like whole grains - brown rice, oats or millets and healthier alternatives to sugar. If you are someone who eats even without any hunger, it's time to wake up to the power of portion control. Be mindful of portions to avoid overeating, which can lead to weight gain and blood sugar spikes.

DIET

- Avoid simple carbohydrates and prefer complex carbohydrates

- Small frequent meals..eating every 2-3 hours

- Adequate protein diet and moderation of oily foods

- Adequate hydration

- Medications and Insulin to be optimised with regular inputs and physician consult.

TO AVOID

- Direct sweets and sugars

- REFINED FLOUR TREATS(MAIDA)

- SUGARY DRINKS AND CARBONATED BEVERAGES

- EEP-FRIED FOODS

- Packaged foods

- QUIT SMOKING

2. Do regular physical exercise

Exercise is a cornerstone of diabetes management. Getting regular physical activity is very important for good health. Exercise makes the body more sensitive to insulin, which helps lower blood sugar levels. Exercise makes the body more sensitive to insulin, which helps lower blood sugar levels and can also help lower high blood pressure and improve cholesterol levels. If you are physically active and exercise for the recommended time, it will help you control weight and improve insulin sensitivity. Aim for at least 150 minutes of moderate-intensity aerobic exercise or 75 minutes of vigorous activity per week. You must choose workout of your choice be it walking, cycling, dancing, or swimming. Including strength training in your workout regime is also important as building muscle can enhance your metabolism and help regulate blood sugar levels.

3. Manage your weight

Being overweight or obese significantly increases the risk of type 2 diabetes. Losing even a small amount of weight can make a big difference. For a person who is overweight or has obesity, a typical goal is to lose 5 to 10 percent of their body weight. Losing even more weight can sometimes reduce the blood sugars to the normal range. Set achievable weight loss goals and seek support from a healthcare professional or a registered dietitian.

4. Monitor your blood sugar

Regularly monitoring your blood sugar levels can help identify any potential issues early. It also helps to understanding how your body responds to food, exercise, and medication. Work closely with your healthcare team to determine the appropriate testing frequency and learn to interpret the results. If you have a family history of diabetes or other risk factors, discuss a screening schedule with your healthcare provider. Today we have continuous glucose monitoring sensors which can give you a complete picture of glucose levels throughout the day. Understanding your blood sugar patterns will enable you to make informed decisions about your diet, exercise, and medication.

5.Medication Adherence

If prescribed by your healthcare provider, taking medications as directed is crucial for managing diabetes effectively. Understand the importance of your medications, their dosage, and potential side effects. If you have concerns or difficulties with your medications, discuss them openly with your healthcare team to find suitable alternatives.

6. Manage your stress

Chronic stress can contribute to the development of diabetes. Explore stress-reduction techniques such as meditation, yoga, deep breathing exercises like pranayama or hobbies to promote relaxation and emotional well-being.

7. Sleep properly

Sleep plays a crucial role in managing diabetes. Not sleeping enough disrupts hormonal balance and can lead to insulin resistance. Strive for 6-8 hours of quality sleep each night to support your overall health. Establish a consistent sleep routine, create a comfortable sleep environment, and avoid stimulants like caffeine close to bedtime.

Preventing diabetes is within your grasp through proactive lifestyle changes. Embracing a balanced diet, regular exercise, weight management, and other healthy habits can significantly reduce your risk of developing this chronic condition. By incorporating these lifestyle modifications into your daily routine, you can effectively manage your diabetes, improve your overall quality of life, and work towards a healthier, more balanced future. Always consult with your healthcare team for personalised advice and guidance tailored to your unique needs.

Chapter 3

Governing Blood Sugar

Step Up to Manage Blood-Sugar Levels

Diabetes is a chronic lifestyle condition that needs to be managed properly to lessen the risk of other health problems in the future. India is currently witnessing an alarming rise of diabetes. Over 101 million Indians are currently living with diabetes. This metabolic disease cannot be fully cured but can be managed with some basic lifestyle changes. Always checking for the sweet value of food before eating, ensuring proper monitoring of blood sugar, regular insulin checks etc, can be a lot for people living with diabetes. Eventually, it does become a lifestyle. And it is only with lifestyle ways that we can keep a check on our body. In particular during Summers, heat exhaustion, heat stroke etc are on a rise. And for people with diabetes,it probably is a time to be a extra cautious with season change. Speaking of health in Summer, people living with diabetes need to be a little more cautious than usual. As temperatures rise during the summer months, it's important to be mindful of the impact that extreme heat can have on your diabetes management. Maintaining blood sugar levels under the sun becomes a task than usual as the temperatures affect glucose levels for diabetic patients more easily. For working professionals, many of whom are doing desk jobs, this can be challenging. Often, the hustling work culture makes us live a more sedentary lifestyle. We are glued to our screens for, keep sitting in one position for a long duration, increase screen time and much more. To fuel your career ambitions and professional growth, good health plays a key role. Health shouldn't hold anyone back professionally. One of the most growing health conditions today that people need to manage effectively including in the workplace - is diabetes.Sometimes making a plan and following it can help us sort out the clutter and indulge a disciplined way to take care of ourselves and for people with diabetes, having a little routine can help regulate the blood sugar levels. With careful planning, you can keep your blood sugar levels in check, so you continue to be at your best throughout the work, day and Night and beyond.

As a result, people living with diabetes are sometimes inconsistent with their lifestyle changes and don't take their medicines as prescribed. It is critical for people with diabetes to take necessary steps to effectively manage their diabetes and properly follow the treatment schedule for better health outcomes."

Routine Ways to Manage Blood Sugar

1. **Have a diabetes action plan that suits your work life:** Navigating your diabetes and work journey starts even before you reach the office. Getting good sleep at night matters as does how you plan for the day. Create a routine so you don't skip breakfast which is important to keep sugar highs and lows at bay. Decide whether you want to have this meal at home or when you get to work but keep

it nutritious. Limit empty calories and cut back on salt and saturated fat.

2. **Stick to your medication routine:** To manage your diabetes well, adhering to medication is important, which helps maintain glycemic control. In case you need to take any medication at work, be sure to set reminders maybe on your phone or with a post-it note on your desk.

3. **Get moving:** Many at work have sedentary lifestyles. Physical activity helps people with diabetes manage their condition better. Get active by stretching at your desk, taking short walks around the office, up and down the stairs, or even outside. A recent study found that a post-meal walk also helps lower your blood sugar levels. Further, try fitting exercise into your routine before or after work.

4. **Learn to manage stress:** When you are stressed, you may notice your glucose levels changing. Sometimes, you may be overwhelmed at work. Good coping mechanisms help keep your blood sugar levels in check when things get difficult. Try meditating in a quiet corner, find time to unwind (talk to a colleague or take a break), and identify and manage stressors.

5. **Healthy Lunch Matters:** Pack lunch smartly so you can enjoy a healthy, balanced meal and aren't only dependant on outside food. A diabetes-friendly diet includes leafy greens (like spinach), non-starchy vegetables (like carrots, tomatoes, onions, okra, cauliflower), healthy carbs (like whole grains and brown rice), lean proteins (including eggs, beans, and chicken), and fruits low in carbohydrates

(such as oranges). On days with special events, whether a colleague's birthday or team lunch, watch your calorie intake beforehand.

Things To Do - Manage Glucose Levels Efficiently

After sleeping for an adequate amount of time, there are days when one wakes up with increased glucose levels during the early morning hours. This is witnessed more in diabetic people and can become a part of their lifestyle. But why does this happen? There may be multiple reasons behind high glucose levels in the morning but one of them could be the 'dawn phenomenon.' The dawn phenomenon occurs early in the morning from 3 am to 8 am, while you are asleep.

Though the cause of this phenomenon is not clear, some researchers believe that the release of certain hormones overnight increases blood sugar levels. This sudden boost in blood sugar level can also take place for reasons like:

– Eating unhealthy or wrong snacks before sleeping.

– Not having enough insulin in your body, the night before, and

– Irregularity with prescribed medicines.

Millions of people are affected by high blood sugar and have now become a lifestyle disease rather than a health disease. However, the effects of the rise in blood sugar levels can differ from person to person. People with high blood sugar should take precautions, especially while eating.

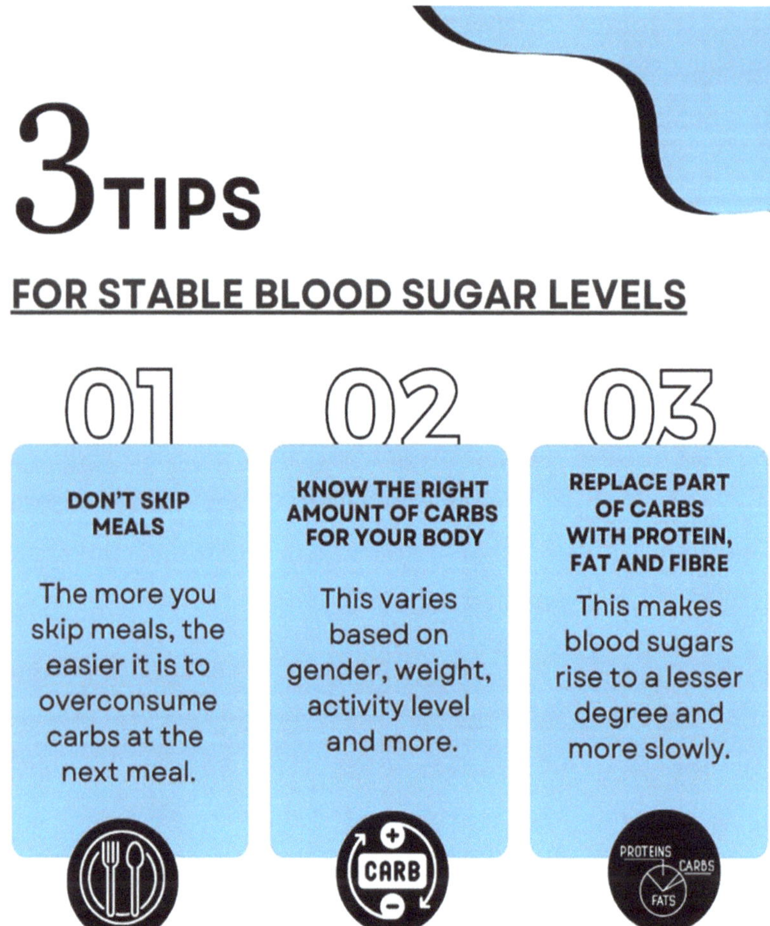

Ways to control high blood sugar levels in the morning:

Diabetic patients should never skip their breakfast. Skipping breakfast can lead to increased hunger and overeating. It can cause an increase in blood sugar. In order to keep your blood sugar under control, you have to give more attention in your breakfast. Because in most people, blood sugar levels raises after breakfast.

Let's see what can be done in the morning to prevent this.

Protein

Eat protein and healthy fats in the morning. For this, it's better to include eggs, Greek yogurt, meat etc in your diet.

Low glycemic index foods

Include low glycemic index foods. Replace refined grains with something like oatmeal in your morning diet.

Sugar and carbohydrates

Try to eat less of these: refined, highly processed carbohydrate foods and those with added sugar. These include sugary drinks like soda, sweet tea and juice, refined grains like white bread, white rice and sugary cereal, and sweets and snack foods like cake, cookies, candy and chips.

Fiber

A high fiber foods is vital for people with diabetes. iber is your friend because it helps with blood sugar control and weight management. It can also lower your risk of heart include more fiber rich foods like Avocado, chia seeds, raspberries etc in your breakfast.

Cinnamon and Fenugreek

Include cinnamon and Fenugreek in your morning diet. It helps to reduce your blood sugar spike.

Water

Drinking enough water is especially important for people with diabetes. Water will not raise blood glucose levels, which is why it is so beneficial to drink when people with diabetes have high blood sugar, as it enables more glucose to be flushed out of the blood.

Regular Exercise

Exercising regularly can be beneficial in controlling the rise in levels of blood sugar in the morning. Walks and other exercises can help in controlling high blood sugar levels. It further helps you maintain weight and can give you a healthy lifestyle.

Take Proper Meals on Time

Proper meals on time are essential to maintain blood sugar levels in individuals, especially for people with diabetes who often experience fluctuations in blood glucose levels. Hence, breakfast, which is the first meal of the day, should be healthy and on time. Eating a balanced breakfast which is low in carbohydrates and high in protein content, fiber-rich fruits, or vegetables can help in maintaining sugar levels.

Keep a Check on your Sugar Level Before Going to bed and Stay Hydrated

Check your blood sugar level before sleeping, if your blood sugar level is high before bedtime then it will remain high throughout the night and hence you will wake up with an elevated level of blood sugar. Further, keep yourself hydrated and drink plenty of water to maintain your blood sugar level.

Bed Time Routine to Maintain Glucose Level

1. **Avoid Late Night Snacking:** It is best to avoid late-night snacks to manage glucose levels. While it is also subjective

to food choice, there are chances to wake up to increase glucose in the morning.

2. **Chamomile tea** (1 cup) - According to Nutritionist Lovneet Batra, these few steps may help with diabetes. Known for its strong astringent, anti-inflammatory and antioxidant properties which significantly optimize blood sugar control.

3. **7 soaked almonds** - Magnesium and tryptophan helps in improving sleep quality, keep night hunger pangs at bay and reduce night time sugar cravings.

4. 1 **tsp soaked methi dan**a - The excellent hypoglycaemic property of fenugreek seeds plays a noteworthy role in alleviating the blood sugar levels of the body.

Chapter 4

DIET - A Key To Your Well-Being

Change in Diet is the most acceptable conventional treatment and prevention for Type 2 Diabetes. To keep the body Healthy, excersise and physical activity along with a strict diet plan with discipline is very necessary.

Moderation Is Ideal Diet Discipline

In the last few years during PANDEMIC, I have lost at least 8 to 9 people known to me personally, and a few celebrities too, who were in their 40s who died because of doing too much to be "fit". Unfortunately they only looked fit, and nothing more than that.

In anything in life, MODERATION is the mantra. Any extreme of zero or 100 is not correct. A moderate amount of exercise, just about 20mins, eating everything, no detoxification or keto moto diets, just eat what your ancestors have been eating, the local and seasonal food in your hometown, not kale, kiwi or olive oil..., but in small quantities, sleeping a full 7 hours, respecting your body is all that you need to do.

It's okay for people with diabetes to eat fat, and to replace spiky carbs with foods that contain fat. That said, some types of fat are healthier than others. We recommend limiting saturated fats and replacing them with unsaturated fats, such as those found in the Mediterranean diet. In practice, this means eating more olive oil, nuts, seeds, avocado, and oily fish, and moderating the amounts meat and dairy.

Nutrition guidelines generally recommend 130 grams of carbohydrates per day for adults without diabetes, but there's no consensus for people with diabetes. diaTribe recommends 100-150 grams per day, which is about 25-30% of a person's daily calories that should come from carbs. This means that if you aim to eat 1,500 calories per day, then about 450 of those calories should come from carbs. We've found that it's easier to stay in range if we limit carbs to 30 grams per meal or snack. You'll have to experiment and find what's right for you and your lifestyle. Counting carbs is the only way to have some idea of how many carbs you consume at each meal. Foods that are low in carbs – such as nuts and dairy products – often contain protein and healthy fats. Some foods have no carbs, because they are primarily made of protein (meats, fish, or eggs) or fat (butter or oils). Low-carb foods are those which usually have little effect on blood sugar. "Slow carbs," on the other hand, are broken down more slowly in the body and have a more predictable effect on blood sugar levels. Slow carbs include veggies that grow above the ground (like leafy greens, broccoli, tomatoes, and cabbage), beans, and fruit (in moderation).

- Foods high in fiber can help prevent glucose spikes. Fiber is a helpful nutrient found in plant foods (vegetables, fruits, beans, and whole grains) that can slow carbohydrate digestion and help manage blood sugar levels.

- Understanding portion size is important for all types of food and can help you make sure you are eating a balanced diet.

- Build colorful meals to make sure you are getting a wide variety of nutrients. Filling your plate with foods of different colors means a focus on eating lots of veggies and some fruit.

- Drink water to keep your body hydrated.

Just eat all that you ate growing up, in small quantities, exercise for 20mins to 30mins...just a good walk should do perfectly and stop all supplements.... Anything but in moderation. Add a bit of silent meditation to your routine.Most importantly, listen to your body. Understand it.

By 40 the body is undergoing a lot of changes, 50 even more, 60 plus your body is starting to slow down, 70 plus, your body is starting to shut down, 80 plus every year is a bonus. So, stop saying 60 is the new 40, 50 is the new 30...no it isn't, if you are 40 or 50 plus, be grateful if you're healthy, slow down so your heart can keep pace, understand retirement has been suggested for a reason, your body and mind cannot take the stress which you once endured. Outwardly you could be looking good, thank your genes but inside, the organs are aging.

If you're 40 + read the above and if you're doing something other than the above, change it, now!! I'm sure you don't want to end up as another statistic.

Power of Portion (Portion Control)

ENGAGING in regular meals and adhering to a balanced diet has become a daily norm. However, the current trend is to randomly adopt diets showcased in online videos in pursuit of health and fitness. Do these routines truly benefit us? The key lies in of then overlooked portion control, sometimes following unsuitable dietary patterns. To dispel this confusion, we sought in sights from experts shedding light on the significance of portion control.

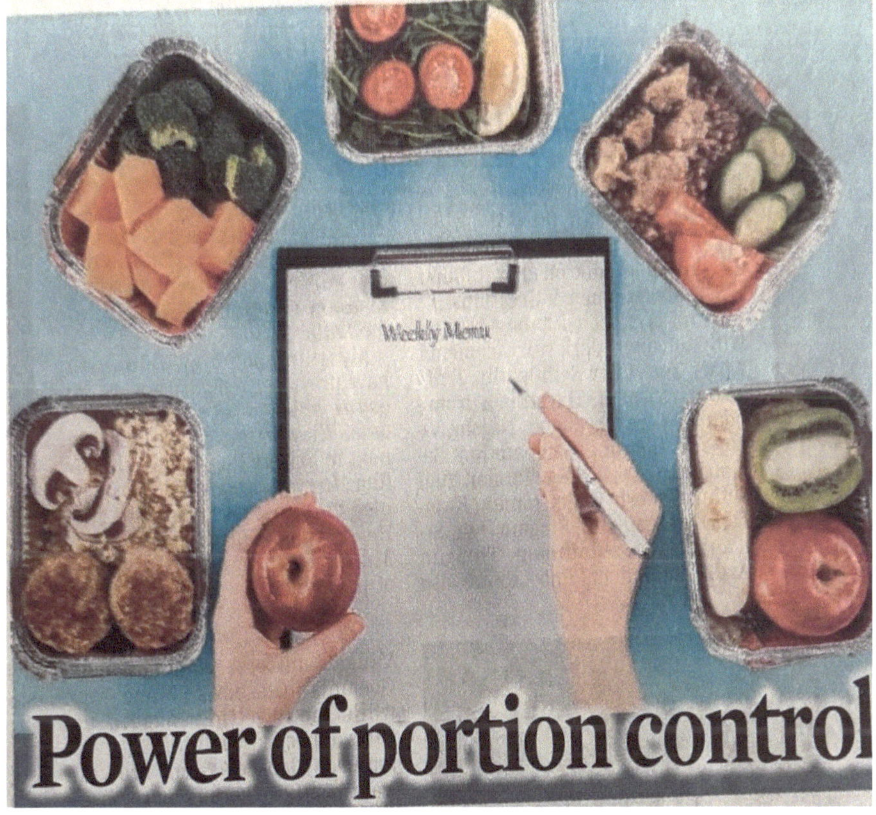

A beautiful Hadiths of Prophet (SAW)on Portion Control Miqdam bin Ma'dikarib (RA) said: "I heard the Messenger of Allah (ﷺ) saying: 'The human does not fill any container that is worse than his stomach. It is sufficient for the son of Adam to eat what will support his back. If this is not possible, then a third for food, a third for drink, and third for his breath."

This is the best diet to follow! One third of your stomach should be full of food, so don't overeat. One third should be reserved for water to allow your body to be nourished, free from toxins and cleansed appropriately. One third for air because we've all felt the pangs of overeating where even breathing and the stomach expanding to draw in oxygen causes discomfort, signalling we have eaten too much. Enjoy food and thank God for it, but look after your body too because you need it to take care of your family and maintain your worship of God. May Allah bless us all with good health.

–Ameen!

A Senior clinical dietician, Care Hospitals, Hyderabad. Emphasizes the importance of portion control and its integration into diets. "Initially, portion control was discussed primarily for diabetic individuals. Focusing on regulating carb intake – replacing simple carbs with complex ones and specifying appropriate quantities within a 1,500-calorie daily limit. Each meal was structured, emphasizing portion control: for instance, two phulkas (Roti) with vegetable salad, a bowl of protein like lentils, vegetable curry, or non-vegetarian items. Gradually, portion control extended beyond diabetic care to weight management. It revolves around selecting healthy quantities of various foods. For instance recommending fruits comes with a caveat of portion sizes – typically 50 to 100 grams per day for diabetics. Vegetables, however, have no such restrictions, encouraging five to six servings. This approach ensures optimal nutrient intake, preventing overconsumption and proving immensely beneficial."

"Initially intended for diabetics, the significance of portion control amplifies, Whether it`s weight gain or reduction. Its tailor-made accordingly. For weight gain, a protein – rich diet with balanced carbs is recommended, incorporating 50 to 100 grams of chicken or paneer, accompanied by ample vegetables and one or two phulkas. Conversely, for weight loss, the emphasis shifts to vegetables, salads, and proteins, with carbs consumed last. Its meticulously divided in food groups based on their portion sizes, aligning with goals like weight regulation or cholesterol control, effectively catering to individual needs.

Regarding the meals to consume for a person on diet, "Instructing individuals on portion control involves advocating smaller plates to reduce calorie intake, This psychological trick makes It appear like a substantial meal, satiating the mind subconsciously, steer away from simple carbs like refined flour, rice and sugar, favouring complex carbohydrates such as, oats, and barley. As for dietary guidelines, especially for diabetic individuals, its recommended small, frequent meals, discouraging overeating and prolonged gaps between meals. The meal plan typically includes breakfast, a moderate lunch and dinner. Additionally, we suggest intermittent snacks like soup, porridge, and green tea, Employing measuring tips – using hand sizes as serving guides, considering palm and fist sizes – helps individuals grasp portion control effectively. The rule of thumb is to allocate half the plate to vegetables (salads, curries, boiled veggies), a quarter for carbs, and the remaining quarter for protein. By employ plate and palm sizes as visual aids, its to facilitate comprehensive understanding of portion control."

Another senior dietician, whom I consulted. Elucidates the essence of portion control. " It involves consuming the right foods in appropriate quantities from each food group, ensuring a safe intake of nutrients while maintaining a balanced calorie count. Prescribing measures based on calorie in-take allows for a harmonious blend of essential nutrients."

Food Hygiene:

Food hygiene have never been more important than the time of Covid19 Pandemic. Safe Food is a shared responsibility & requires joint efforts. let's spread awareness about food safety, good eating habits & hygiene practices in order to prevent food borne illness.

Food Hygiene, otherwise known as Food Safety can be defined as handling, preparing and storing food or drink in a way that best reduces the risk of consumers becoming sick from the food-borne disease. The principles of food safety aim to prevent food from becoming contaminated and causing **food poisoning.**

5 Food Safety Rules In The Kitchen:

- **Rule 1:** Wash hands between steps. ...

- **Rule 2:** Sanitize work surfaces. ...

- **Rule 3:** Use separate cutting boards for raw meats, vegetables and produce, and cooked foods. ...

- **Rule 4:** Cook foods to safe temperatures. ...

- **Rule 5:** Keep hot foods hot and cold foods cold. ...

Chapter 5

The Impact of Food on Health and Well-Being

Purnima Varghese an expert in Diabetes Care and Management states in one of her article that Diabetes is a chronic condition which can be managed with healthy eating. The main goal of food is to maintain your sugar level and not cause excessive spikes and falls.

Fibre is an essential part of a healthy diet, and it is important to include a variety of high-fibre foods in your daily meals. A high-fibre diet can help to promote digestive health, control blood sugar levels, and reduce the risk of heart disease, stroke, and other chronic conditions.

A Good Source of Fibre

Let's explore some of the foods that are highest in fibre.

1. **Beans and legumes**

   Beans and legumes are some of the most fibre-rich foods available. They are also a good source of protein, making them an excellent choice for vegetarians and vegans. Examples of fibre-rich bueans and legumes include chickpeas, lentils, black beans, kidney beans, and navy beans. One cup of cooked beans can provide up to 15 grams of fibre.

2. Whole grains

Whole grains are another excellent source of fibre. They are also a good source of complex carbohydrates, which can provide sustained energy throughout the day. Examples of whole grains include brown rice, quinoa, bulgur, barley, and whole wheat pasta. One cup of cooked whole grains can provide up to 8 grams of fibre. They have a low glycemic index as compared to processed carbohydrates. They are also very high in fibre, which prevents glucose from entering the bloodstream too quickly.

Brown rice contains lots of vitamins, minerals, and fiber. It has lower glycemic index that can reduce the incidence of diabetes.

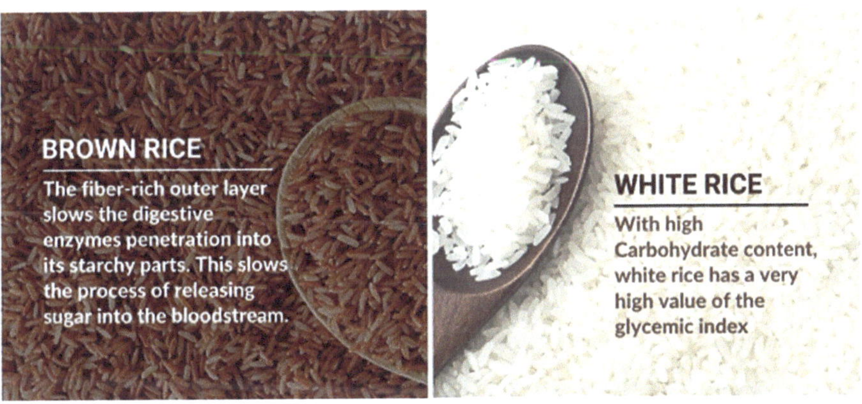

3. Fruits

Fruits are a delicious and healthy way to add fibre to your diet. They are also a good source of vitamins and minerals.

Some of the most fibre-rich fruits include apples, pears, berries, oranges, and bananas. One medium-sized fruit can provide up to 4 grams of fibre. When choosing fruits, choose ones with a lower glycemic index (GI), as they have a softer effect on blood sugar these are the fruits that can help control blood sugar levels, making them excellent choices for individuals looking to manage their sugar intake. There is also a group of low-sugar fruits that are suitable for managing diabetes. All fruits, of course, have higher nutrient and fibre content than processed foods with added sugar. Your blood sugar won't surge as rapidly after eating fruit since high-fibre meals slow down digestion. However, you may not be aware of the amount of sugar that fruit contains. Perhaps you have diabetes and are interested in learning which fruits will affect your blood sugar levels the least.

What makes apples so great for diabetics is that while they do contain sugar the type of sugar they contain is mostly fructose, which causes only a small rise in blood sugar when eaten as a fruit. Apples also contain fibre that slows the absorption of sugar into the bloodstream.

4. **Vegetables**

Vegetables are another excellent source of fibre. They are also low in calories and high in vitamins and minerals. Some of the most fibre-rich vegetables include Oakra (Bhendi) broccoli, Brussels sprouts, artichokes, spinach, and sweet potatoes. One cup of cooked vegetables can provide up to 6 grams of fibre.

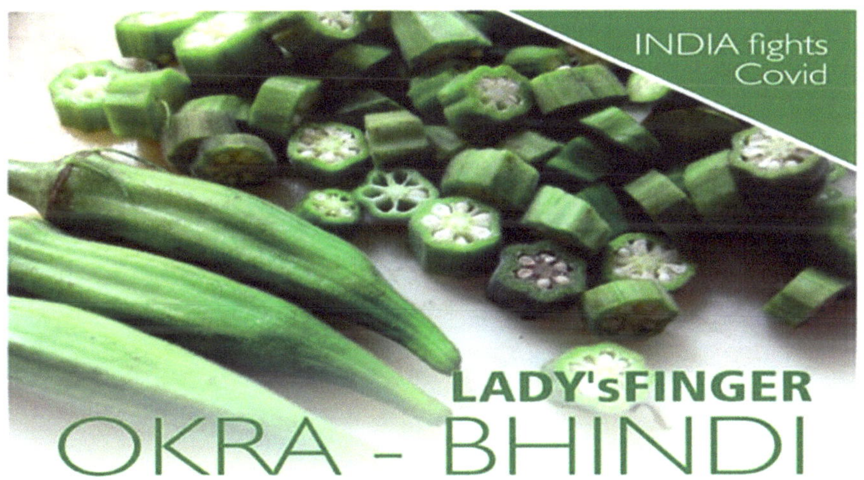

OKRA – BHINDI

Bhindi, a rare **Protein rich** green vegetable pod is available all across the country in Summers. With Covid simmering, this is one of the best bet for diabetics.

Take two pieces of lady's finger, cut both ends and make a small cut in the middle of the pod. Put both in a glass of water and keep it overnight at room temperature. Drink **just the water** before the breakfast and do this regularly for two weeks and see for yourself ....the dramatic normalization of your blood sugar levels.

Infusion of **roasted Okra seeds** has long been practised in Turkey for Diabetes; it has been liked to inhibit intestinal enzyme alpha–glucosidase thus contributing to low sugar absorption.

Thick gel – Mucilage of Okra contains polysaccharide Rhamnogalacturonan which binds with **Fats, Sugar and Cholesterol** thus reducing their absorption by intestines. Mucilage in advanced studies is being touted as complex replacement to human blood plasma. **High dietry fibre** promotes intestinal flora.

Compounds in Bhindi impact the regulation of ALP and AST (liver dysfunction) reducing **insulin resistance.** Soup of Okra has found to be useful in African **HIV patients.**

Bhindi is rich in Vitamin K,A,C,B6, Magnesium, Zinc, Pottasium, Iron, Calcium and antioxidants like **IsoQuercetin.** Linoleic acid in seeds is inhibitor of lipid peroxidation (spoiling of fats in body). **Polyphenols, Flavanoids** lowers risk of blood clots and oxidiative damage of cells.

5. **Nuts and seeds**

Nuts and seeds are not only delicious but also a good source of healthy fats and fibre. Examples of fibre-rich nuts and seeds include almonds, chia seeds, flaxseeds, and pumpkin seeds. A handful of nuts or seeds can provide up to 5 grams of fibre.

6. **Oats**

Oats are a popular breakfast food and are also a good source of fibre. They are also a good source of complex carbohydrates and can help to regulate blood sugar levels. One cup of cooked oats can provide up to 4 grams of fibre.

7. **Dried fruits**

Dried fruits are a convenient and portable way to add fibre to your diet. They are also a good source of vitamins and minerals. Examples of fibre-rich dried fruits include dates, prunes, and figs. One ounce of dried fruit can provide up to 3 grams of fibre.

8. **Popcorn**

Popcorn is a low-calorie and fibre-rich snack. It is also a good source of whole grains. One cup of air-popped popcorn can provide up to 1 gram of fibre.

In conclusion, there are many foods that are high in fibre. Adding these foods to your diet can help to promote digestive health, control blood sugar levels, and reduce the risk of chronic conditions. But do remember everything in Moderation.

The Crucial Role of Protein in Managing Diabetes

The quote **"May you always value the simple little things in life, for they make a big difference and hence are the most** important," resonates when all of us think about well-being and nutrition.

Neelanjana Singh, Nutrition and Wellness consultant believes that it is the simple tweaks with diet that can make a shift towards better health. The simplicity makes it sustainable as well as doable.

"Let me explain this by taking the case of individuals who are diabetic. Studies have confirmed that the consumption of protein rich foods as the first item in the meal helps reduce the spikes in blood sugar. This means consuming dal/curd/raita/paneer/fish/egg first in the meal, followed by the cereals (wheat/millets/rice) in combination with dals/curd/paneer/meat. Several studies have confirmed that increasing protein intake and reducing intake of carbohydrates helps lower HbA1C. This is why the order in which the foods are consumed is critical to maintaining blood glucose levels," adds Singh.

Among the various lifestyle diseases, diabetes is on the rise worldwide and India ranks number two when it comes to the number of diabetics in the world. During the COVID pandemic, most people were homebound, which led to decreased physical activity, increased consumption of unhealthy foods, irregular sleep patterns, and elevated levels of stress, because of which India is witnessing a huge epidemic of diabetes and obesity combined.

When it comes to diabetes management, nutrition forms the cornerstone. "As carbohydrates impact blood glucose levels the most, dietary strategies focus on decreasing consumption of refined/simple carbohydrates and replacing it with complex carbohydrates that are high on fibre. This strategy by itself is not good enough unless it is combined with adequate proteins in the diet," opines Singh.

Protein is often viewed as a big factor in weight management, but there is so much more to it that is often overlooked. This indispensable and versatile nutrient makes up the framework of the body's defense system, enzymes and hormones. It also helps in muscle building, repair of tissues, and aids one to lead an active life. Protein has several other benefits when it comes to people with diabetes.

Adequate protein consumption helps build a robust immune system. "We know that people with diabetes are susceptible to infections as their immune function is compromised. Moreover, people with diabetes are often overweight or obese, hence including protein in adequate amounts helps manage weight by providing the much needed satiety and controlling hunger pangs," adds Singh.

The Indian diet is predominantly low in protein and there are very many studies and surveys to confirm this. In a recent study among 1000 Indian patients with diabetes, only 14.3% participants were consuming adequate protein. Low protein diets along with uncontrolled diabetes can lead to several complications. A poor immune system and loss of muscle mass are two of the many detrimental effects it can have.

Increasing the consumption of protein rich foods amongst people with diabetes is one of my primary objectives as a nutrition therapist. Good sources of protein include milk and milk products, yogurt, cottage cheese, whole pulses, soya, fish, lean meat, which need to be incorporated into all meals as well as snack items. "Simple dietary tweaks can help achieve targets of adequate protein at every meal. For example, blend besan into wheat flour for making chapatis, use beans for making a salad along with greens, try hummus as a spread instead of mayonnaise, make tikkis of channa instead of aloo, and so on. The list of examples is inexhaustible," believes Singh.

Promoting better glycemic control, muscle health and immunity in people with diabetes is possible through simple dietary modifications. A balanced, wholesome diet helps diabetics lead an active and energetic life. Supplements of protein should be considered to fill any gaps in the requirements after a detailed assessment of intake is carried out.

- **Eggs!** Not only are they a wonderful source of protein, but eggs improve insulin sensitivity and blood sugar control while giving your HDL (the good cholesterol) a boost. They also provide antioxidants that protect from eye disease.

  Leafy green vegetables are a great addition to any diet. They also contain lutein, a nutrient that protects against cataracts and macular degeneration, eye diseases that are common in diabetics.

- ***Nuts.** Not only are nuts a tasty snack, but they're actually really nutritious. They're full of fibre and low in digestible carbs. What's more, research has shown that adding nuts to your regular diet can reduce inflammation and lower blood sugar Nuts have also been found to lower insulin levels. This is good to know as type 2 diabetics often have high insulin levels, which are linked to obesity.

– **Flaxseeds** are what's known as a superfood. High in fibre, they have been shown to be helpful in maintaining blood sugar levels and glycemic control.

Several studies have concluded that **cinnamon** can actually lower blood sugar levels and improve insulin sensitivity. just be sure to limit yourself to less than a teaspoon per day.

– **apple cider** vinegar has some interesting health benefits for diabetics. First, it improves your insulin sensitivity. Second, it can lower your blood sugar response by as much as 20 per cent when you eat carbs, according to Health Line.

– **Fatty fish such as salmon, sardines and anchovies** are a great source of DHA and EPA. These omega-3 fatty acids provide major heart health benefits and are super important for diabetics because they are at increased risk of heart disease and stroke.

A **baked sweet potato** will cause your blood. sugar to rise 30 per cent less than eating a white potato. Sweet potatoes are also loaded with soluble fibre that "lowers cholesterol and slows digestion," according to Best Health.

– **lean cuts of chicken and turkey** are low-calorie proteins that are awesome for keeping you full and maintaining consistent blood sugar levels.

Dietary Fructose and Diabetes - Its Metabolic Effects

Fructose, a natural sugar found in fruits and honey, can have different effects on blood sugar levels compared to glucose,

another common sugar. While fructose itself doesn't directly reduce blood sugar levels, its impact on blood sugar regulation is mediated by various factors:

- **Low Glycemic Index:** Fructose has a lower glycemic index (GI) compared to glucose. The GI measures how quickly a carbohydrate-containing food raises blood glucose levels. Foods with a lower GI lead to a slower and more gradual increase in blood sugar.

- **Insulin Response:** Fructose has a minimal effect on insulin secretion compared to glucose. Insulin is a hormone that helps regulate blood sugar levels by facilitating the uptake of glucose into cells. The reduced insulin response to fructose may contribute to a more stable blood sugar profile.

- **Gluconeogenesis Inhibition:** Fructose metabolism occurs primarily in the liver, where it can be converted into glucose through a process called gluconeogenesis. However, fructose has been shown to inhibit its own conversion to glucose, which may contribute to lower blood sugar levels.

It's important to note that while these aspects may suggest a more favorable impact on blood sugar levels, excessive consumption of fructose, especially in the form of added sugars and sweetened beverages, has been associated with metabolic issues, including insulin resistance and elevated triglycerides.

Consuming fructose in its natural form from whole fruits, which also contain fiber and various nutrients, is generally considered healthier than consuming large amounts of added sugars.

As with any dietary component, moderation is key, and individual responses may vary.

Food to Avoid

Refined starches, like white flour and white rice, with low fibre and high Sugar content are to be avoided at all costs. These products have a very high glycemic index that can send a diabetic person's blood sugar soaring. Eating white rice has a glucose-raising effect. It releases sugar very quickly into the bloodstream.

Coffee is fine for diabetics but many of the concoctions found in specialty coffee shops can contain as many calories as a dessert! Try tea instead!

Dried fruits make great snacks; just not for diabetics. They have great fibre content and nutrients, but their dehydrated state makes it easy to eat more than you should, which will make your blood Sugar climb.

Full-fat dairy products can not only raise your LDL cholesterol levels, thereby increasing your risk of heart disease, but they have also been shown to increase insulin resistance.

Char-grilled,the burnt parts of the meat cause damage to the cell membranes and insulin receptors that are linked to insulin resistance,Not That! Be sure to remove any extremely blackened parts before eating.

People with diabetes need to watch out for the glycemic index and also Glycemic Load in the food they consume. Foods that claim low GI help raise blood sugar levels steadily as compared to ones with high glycemic index.Raising blood sugars slowly means the food will keep you fuller for longer. Lets understand these two important terminologies for a better management of our Diabetes.

Glycemic Index

The **glycemic index** (GI) is a value used to measure how much specific foods increase blood sugar levels. Foods are classified as low, medium, or high **glycemic** foods and ranked on a scale of 0–100. The lower the **GI** of a specific food, the less it may affect your blood sugar levels (1).

It gives you an idea about how fast your body converts the carbs in a food into glucose. Two foods with the same amount of carbohydrates can have different **glycemic index** numbers. The smaller the number, the less impact the food has on your blood sugar. 55 or less = Low (good) 56- 69 = Medium.

Low-GI foods (with scores of 55 and under) include oatmeal, peanuts, peas, carrots, kidney beans, hummus, skim milk and most fruits.

Low GI : Green **vegetables**, most fruits, raw carrots, kidney beans, chickpeas, lentils and bran **breakfast cereals**. Medium GI : Sweet corn, bananas, raw pineapple, raisins, oat **breakfast cereals**, and multigrain, oat bran or rye bread. High GI : White rice, **white bread** and potatoes.

Overall, **bananas** score between **low** and medium on the **GI** scale (between 42 to 62, depending on the ripeness) (10). In addition to sugar and starch, **bananas** contain some fiber.

This means that the sugars in **bananas** are more slowly digested and absorbed, which could prevent blood sugar spikes.

Fruits like berries, cherries, apples, and citrus fruits tend to have lower glycemic indexes and can help manage blood sugar levels better compared to high-sugar fruits like watermelon or bananas. However, portion control is still important. Consulting a healthcare professional or a registered dietitian can provide personalized advice for managing sugar intake.

Glycemic Load

The **glycemic load** (GL) of food is a number that estimates how much the food will raise a person's blood glucose level after eating it. One unit of **glycemic load** approximates the effect of eating one gram of glucose.

Glycemic load helps you account for both the quantity and the quality of your carbs at the same time. Less than 10 is low; more than 20 is high. For a diet with a lower **glycemic load**, eat: More whole grains, nuts, legumes, fruits, vegetables without starch, and other foods with a low **glycemic** index.

Foods with a low glycemic load of 10 or less include:

- ¼ cup **peanuts** (GL of 1)

- 8 oz skim milk (GL of 4)

- 2 cups **watermelon** (GL of 4.3)

- 1 cup **kidney beans** (GL of 7)

- 1 cup all bran cereal (GL of 9)

A few Low-Glycemic Fruits for Diabetes.

- Cherries.

- Grapefruit.

- Dried apricots.

- Pears.

- Apples.

- Oranges.

- Plums.

Conclusion

Diabetes is controlled by Diet, Medication or a combination of the two. Here is a quick list of some of the benificial foods for people living with diabetes.

Fruits with Low-Sugar Content for Diabetics

1. **Pomegranate:** It has a low glycemic load (GL) and glycemic index (GI), which is advantageous for people with high blood sugar levels. In addition to having a low sugar content, it also has a lot of antioxidants, vitamins, and minerals, all of which work to lessen insulin resistance.

2. **Oranges:** They can be a component of a diabetes-friendly diet when eaten in moderation as whole fruits. They are a good source of fibre, antioxidants, and vitamin C. Despite the low sugar level, it's still vital to pay attention to portion amounts because they naturally contain sugar.

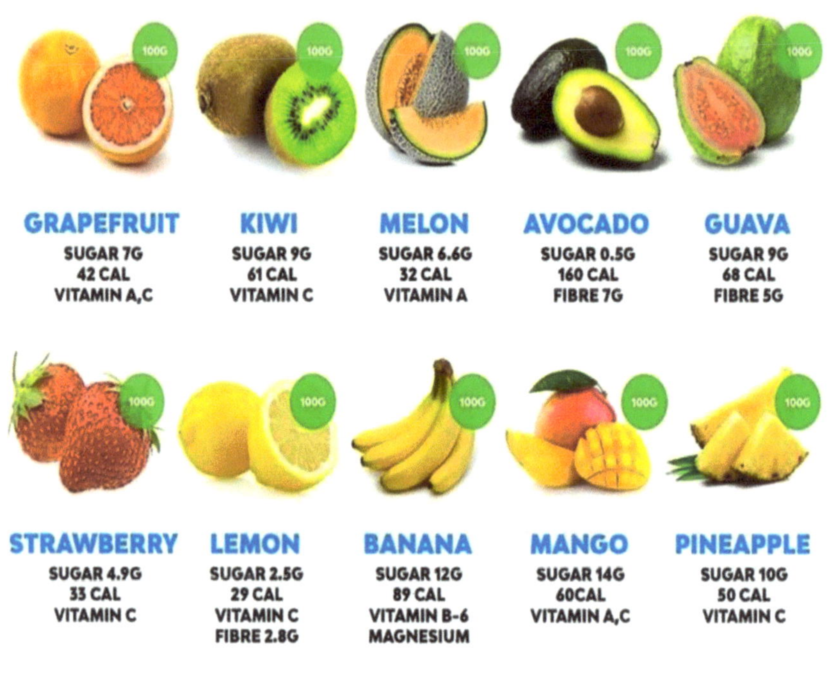

3. **Lemons:** They and their green equivalents are rather acidic fruits that are rich in vitamin C. The average amount of sugar in a lime is 1.13 grams, whereas that in a lemon is 2.1 grams. For a glass of water, they are the ideal tasty, low-sugar complement.

4. **Berries:** In addition to being tasty, berries like strawberries, blueberries, and raspberries also have a very low sugar content. They are abundant in vitamins, fibre, and

antioxidants. They are a great option for those with diabetes since they are low in carbs and have a low glycemic index.

5. **Pears:** They are low in sugar and have soluble fibre, vitamins, and minerals, all of which can help with better blood sugar regulation. They can satiate you and have a low glycemic index, which can help you regulate your sugar needs. Pears' high fibre content increases a sensation of fullness, slows down the absorption of sugar, and helps control blood sugar levels.

As a result, diabetics may still profit from fruits without risking their health by balancing their intake of sugar and vitamins.

List of food items that are beneficial for diabetics and those looking for a healthy lifestyle:

Avocados:

Avocados have healthy fat. Avocados have roughly about 20 types of vitamins and minerals.

Consuming healthy fats keep you full longer.

Walnuts

Walnuts should be your supreme choice as it combines proteins, fibre and healthy fats. Switch your packet of wafers with this and reduce your risk of heart diseases and diabetes.

Seeds like Pumpkin

Pumpkin seeds is high in good fatty acid. Lack of magnesium leads to insulin resistance. Insulin resistance is the leading cause of diabetes.

Pumpkin seeds can be added to salads as dressing or just consumed as a handful.

Chia Seeds

Chia seeds has been trending in general for people of all ages at the moment. Chia seeds is rich in antioxidants, fibre, iron and calcium.

1 ounce chia seeds = 10g fibre.

You can sprinkle this on top of your salad or dessert and achieve that extra crunch.

Ginger

Ginger is anti-inflammatory and can help reduce the risk of diabetes and long term complications. Ginger is known to reduce fasting blood sugar levels in type 2 diabetics. You can add ginger to your tea.

Cinnamon

Cinnamon helps lower blood sugar levels. You can add cinnamon to roasted carrots, or your sweet potatoes. You can even sprinkle some over your tea or milk.

Spinach

Spinach is one of the best sources of potassium. Potassium deficiency has been linked to risk of diabetes and related complications.

One cup banana has 539 milligrams potassium whereas spinach has 839 milligrams.

Tomatoes

Tomatoes are low glycemic index fruits. As per studies, consuming 1 -1.5 medium size tomatoes on a daily basis helps reduce blood pressure. What else? Tomatoes give you good skin.

Oats:

One cup oats = approx. 27g of carbs. This makes oats in a day ideal for your consumption. Oats are also rich in fibre and have low glycemic index.

Beans:

They are the most nutritious food choice as they are high in fibre as well as protein.

In a Nutshell: Eat and Not to Eat

Eat more:	Eat mindfully:	Eat less:
Nutritious foods that often won't affect blood sugar levels	Nutritious foods that may affect your blood sugar and other markers of health	Foods that can spike your blood sugar and harm your health
Non-starchy vegetables, especially green veggies and veggies that grow above ground	Fruit, especially berries Red meat	Sugar and honey Cakes, cookies, ice cream Candy

Nuts and seeds Beans, hummus Soy beans and tofu Eggs Lean protein – chicken and fish Olive oil Avocado Whole grains (such as quinoa, brown rice, and wild rice)	Plain yogurt Dairy products: milk, cheese, cottage cheese, sour cream, and butter Steel cut oatmeal Sweet potato Carrots Sweet corn Whole wheat pasta Low-carb bread products	Sweetened yogurts Regular soda (avoid) Fruit juice (avoid) White rice Bread Potatoes, Crackers Breakfast cereal Chips Dried fruits Processed foods Packaged foods with long ingredient lists

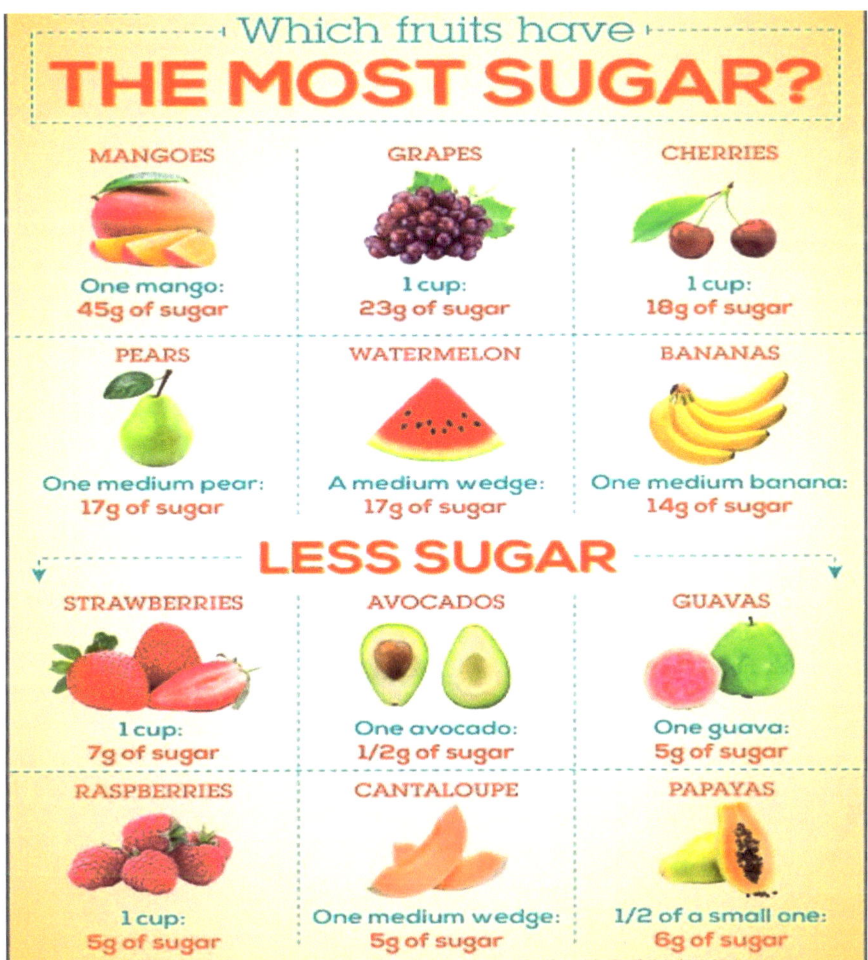
Which fruits have
THE MOST SUGAR?
MANGOES
One mango:
45g of sugar
GRAPES
1 cup:
23g of sugar
CHERRIES
1 cup:
18g of sugar
PEARS
One medium pear:
17g of sugar
WATERMELON
A medium wedge:
17g of sugar
BANANAS
One medium banana:
14g of sugar
LESS SUGAR
STRAWBERRIES
1 cup:
7g of sugar
AVOCADOS
One avocado:
1/2g of sugar
GUAVAS
One guava:
5g of sugar
RASPBERRIES
1 cup:
5g of sugar
CANTALOUPE
One medium wedge:
5g of sugar
PAPAYAS
1/2 of a small one:
6g of sugar

Chapter 6

Exercise- Physical Activity....... A Key to healthy Lifestyle

This year's study by The Indian Council of Medical Research (ICMR) showed that over 100 million people are suffering from this lifestyle disorder in India, and another 136 million are prediabetic. In type 2 diabetes, a person is either unable to produce enough insulin for energy or it doesn't use the insulin produced for energy. The symptoms include increased thirst, frequent urination, hunger, fatigue and blurred vision. In some cases, there may be no symptoms.

Managing your diet, exercise, medication and insulin therapy are the treatments available for it. Though it is a chronic progressive disease, it is reversible.

Does Exercise help for low Blood Sugar?

To keep the body healthy, exercise and Physical Activity are very necessary. In fact, people who have diabetes also have to exercise regularly. With exercise, the blood sugar levels of diabetics will be relatively stable.

So, if you are at risk of developing diabetes, or have type 1 and type 2 diabetes, exercise can provide benefits.

The American College of Sports Medicine and the American Diabetes Association agree that exercise is important for optimal health in diabetics. When we exercise, the body burns glucose or blood sugar as fuel. This process helps lower blood sugar levels.

Walking:

There have been several studies about the health benefits of walking, especially brisk walking. A recent study now shows that walking faster can actually lower the risk of developing type 2 diabetes, and manage your blood sugar levels.

While walking is shown to reduce the risk of type 2 Diabetes, the new study emphasises the pace at which you're doing this exercise.

Researchers, who published the study on Nov'23 in the British Journal of Sports Medicine, found that walking fast can lower the risk of diabetes by 40%.

The study authors reviewed 10 previous studies conducted between 1999 and 2022. They assessed the links between walking speed and the development of type 2 diabetes among adults from the United States, the United Kingdom and Japan.

Walking at a leisurely or relaxed pace was categorised as below 3.2 kilometres per hour.

A standard or typical speed fell within the range of 3.2 to 4.8 kilometres per hour. A pace described as "fairly brisk" ranged from 4.8 to 6.4 kilometres per hour. Walking at brisk/striding pace exceeded 6.4 Km /hr. Every kilometre increase in walking speed beyond brisk was linked to a 9% decrease in the risk of developing the disease.

The study affirms the idea that intensity is important for the prevention of diabetes.

Those who walked at a speed of higher than 6 kilometers per hour had a 39% lower risk of developing the condition.

"While current strategies to increase total walking time are beneficial, it may also be reasonable to encourage people to walk at faster speeds to further increase the health benefits of walking," researchers said.

HIIT (High Intensity Interval Training):

High-intensity interval training, HIIT for short, is a workout involving brief bursts of activity with active recovery periods. Because of the intensity, the workouts are short, which is appealing for those who are pressed for time.

As the name "high-intensity" implies, you push yourself hard during those bursts.

Is it Safer People with Diabetes to do HIIT?

Studies have shown that not only is HIIT usually safe for people with diabetes, but it may be an option for those with a tight schedule or a fear of Hypoglycemia.

Before jumping into a HIIT workout, there are special considerations, especially if you're taking insulin or other glucose-lowering medications. That, and everyone responds differently to exercise.

"While using a HIIT program can show benefits to blood sugar management by burning glucose and improving insulin sensitivity.

"HIIT would be best for those with stable blood sugar levels and who have been cleared to participate in moderate to intense exercise. If you have diabetes and are looking to add HIIT to your workout routine, it's always a good idea to consult with your healthcare team to ensure it's a safe option for them.

Sample HIIT exercises

The great thing about HIIT is its versatility. It can also be done at home or in a gym. You can perform HIIT exercises with your body weight, dumbbells, kettlebells, treadmill, bike, rowing machine, bands, or the elliptical.

Here are a few examples of a HIIT workout:

- Jump rope for 30 seconds and rest for 30 seconds; repeat as many times as possible.

- Kettlebell swings for 10 minutes; swing for 45 seconds, rest for 15 seconds.

- Dumbbell squats for 20 seconds, rest for 10 seconds; repeat until you can't do it anymore.

- Burpees (exercise where you squat, do a pushup, and then jump in the air) for 20 seconds, rest for 30 seconds; 10 rounds.

- Pushups for 30 seconds, rest for 10 seconds; six rounds.

- Sprint on treadmill for 12 minutes; run for 20 seconds, rest for 30 seconds.

- Brisk walk for 40 seconds, slow down for 40 seconds; repeat for 20 minutes.

Benefits of HIIT for diabetes

Besides saving time and adding variety to your physical activity routine, HIIT has multiple benefits for someone with diabetes.

Glucose control

HIIT sessions have a greater glucose-lowering effect when compared to walking on a treadmill. Improved blood sugar levels aren't just for the young, either – HIIT also improves blood sugar in older adults.

Improved body composition

Resistance exercises like weight lifting promote muscle growth, but HIIT may also give you gains. HIIT increase muscle capacity. thereby increasing muscle mass. Along with muscle growth, HIIT may also reduce body fat percentage.

The reduction in body mass index, waist circumference, and body fat are similar and sometimes better with HIIT when compared to moderate-intensity continuous exercise.

Insulin sensitivity

Regular exercise can improve insulin sensitivity over time. This means that the body becomes more efficient at using insulin to transport glucose into cells, potentially reducing the overall need for insulin.

At the same time, HITT can initially lead to an increase in insulin requirements. This is because the body may require more glucose to fuel muscles during activity. Responses to exercise can vary among individuals.

Chapter 7

The Two Subordinates of Diabetes - Cholestrol & Obesity

Diabetes damages the lining of your arteries. This means it's more likely that cholesterol will stick to them, making them narrow or even blocked. If you have diabetes, you will usually have lower levels of HDL (good) cholesterol and higher levels of LDL/non-HDL (bad) cholesterol.

Obesity, particularly when associated with increased abdominal and intra-abdominal fat distribution and increased intrahepatic and intramuscular triglyceride content, is a major risk factor for prediabetes and type 2 diabetes because it causes both insulin resistance and β-cell dysfunction.

The accumulation of an excessive amount of body fat can cause type 2 diabetes, and the risk of type 2 diabetes increases linearly with an increase in Body Mass Index (BMI). Accordingly, the worldwide increase in the prevalence of obesity has led to a concomitant increase in the prevalence of type 2 diabetes. Obesity and type 2 diabetes share a close association. Research highlights that obesity is a common risk factor that can lead to the development of prediabetes and type 2 diabetes. Maintaining a moderate weight and making certain lifestyle adjustments can help slow or prevent diabetes. Some evidence indicates that an individual with obesity is approximately

10 times more likely to develop type 2 diabetes than someone with a moderate body weight.

Carrying extra weight raises your chances of having too much low-density lipoprotein (LDL), or "bad cholesterol," in your blood. That raises your chances of heart problems and other serious issues. Every 10 pounds you're overweight causes your body to produce as much as 10 milligrams of extra cholesterol every day.

What causes high cholesterol

Cholesterol is a fatty substance found in the blood that is necessary for various bodily functions, such as the production of hormones and the formation of cell membranes. However, when cholesterol levels become too high, it can lead to health problems, particularly cardiovascular disease.

There are two main types of cholesterol: Low Density Lipoprotein (LDL) & High Density Liopoprotein (HDL).

LDL cholesterol is often referred to as "bad" cholesterol because it tends to accumulate in the arteries, forming plaques that can restrict blood flow.

HDL cholesterol, on the other hand, is considered "good" cholesterol as it helps remove excess cholesterol from the bloodstream and prevents plaque buildup.

Several factors contribute to high cholesterol levels:

- **Diet:** Consuming foods high in saturated and trans fats can increase LDL cholesterol levels. These unhealthy fats are commonly found in red meat, full-fat dairy products, fried foods, and processed snacks. A diet rich in fruits, vegetables, whole grains, and lean proteins, on the other hand, can help maintain healthy cholesterol levels.

- **Obesity:** Being overweight or obese can raise LDL cholesterol levels and lower HDL cholesterol levels. Excess body fat, particularly around the waist, can lead to increased cholesterol production in the liver.

- **Lack of physical activity:** Regular exercise has been shown to increase HDL cholesterol levels and improve overall cardiovascular health. Leading a sedentary lifestyle can contribute to higher LDL cholesterol levels.

- **Smoking:** Smoking damages blood vessels, lowers HDL cholesterol, and increases LDL cholesterol. It also increases the risk of other cardiovascular diseases, making it a significant risk factor for high cholesterol.

- **Genetics:** In some cases, high cholesterol levels can be inherited. Familial hypercholesterolemia is a genetic condition that causes very high LDL cholesterol levels and increases the risk of early heart disease.

- **Age and gender:** Cholesterol levels tend to rise with age, particularly in women after menopause. Prior to menopause, estrogen helps maintain higher levels of HDL cholesterol. After menopause, however, HDL cholesterol levels may decrease, contributing to increased overall cholesterol levels.

- **Certain medical conditions:** Conditions such as diabetes, hypothyroidism, kidney disease, and liver disease can affect cholesterol metabolism and lead to elevated cholesterol levels.

It is important to note that high cholesterol levels often do not cause any symptoms, which is why regular cholesterol screenings are recommended, especially for individuals with risk factors. Lifestyle modifications, such as adopting a healthy diet, engaging in regular physical activity, quitting smoking, and maintaining a healthy weight, are typically the first line of treatment for high cholesterol. In some cases, medication may be prescribed to help manage cholesterol levels effectively. It is always advisable to consult with a healthcare professional for personalized advice and guidance based on your specific health situation.

10 Weight Loss tips for obese people:

COOK IN COCONUT OIL: Coconut oil is said to be rich in special fats that boost metabolism. Beware, don't add it to what you're already eating, replace your cooking fats with coconut oil.

EAT EGGS FOR BREAKFAST: Any source of quality protein for breakfast can do the trick, but whole eggs can help you eat fewer calories for the next 36 hours, and lose more body fat.

DON'T DRINK SUGARY JUICES: Cut down on your intake of coke bottles and packaged juices with added sugar.

MUNCH ON HEALTHY FOODS: Keep nuts and dry fruits handy for the times when you feel hungry instead of going for fatty foods.

AEROBIC EXERCISES: Burn calories, improve your physical and mental health with cardio and aerobic exercises.

EAT MORE VEGETABLES AND FRUITS: Eating fruits and vegetables can have many advantages. Not only are they rich in fiber and water, but they also contain few calories. Moreover, it takes time to chew them, which helps to lose weight.

DRINK GREEN TEA: Green tea contains small amounts of caffeine, but it is also loaded with powerful antioxidants that enhance fat burning.

DRINK WATER BEFORE MEALS: Water not only keeps the skin clean and hydrated, but also boosts metabolism and burns calories.

GET GOOD SLEEP: Studies show that poor sleep is one of the strongest risk factors for obesity, being linked to an 89% increased risk of obesity in children, and 55% in adults.

KILL YOUR FOOD ADDICTION: Do you have unwanted food cravings that make you eat more than your metabolism needs? You must seek help and find effective treatment.

Chapter 8

Misconceptions About Diabetes - Know The Facts

Even though diabetes is one of the most widespread health issues in the world, there are still several myths and misconceptions plaguing the condition, creating plenty of confusion among people. There is no shortage of information available about diabetes, but it's essential to remember that not all of it is true. Being aware of this condition is the only way to manage it and prevent any adverse complications. So, here is a list of some of the most common misconceptions surrounding diabetes and the truth behind them.

Myth:

- **I never eat sweets, I can't get diabetes.**

  - **Fact:** Contrary to popular opinion, diabetes is not caused only by eating sweets and sugar-loaded food. In fact, every food we eat is converted into a form of sugar called glucose. A hormone produced by the pancreas, known as insulin, allows the cells to utilise this glucose to function and produce energy. Diabetes occurs when the body is unable to produce sufficient insulin, which results in excess glucose levels in the blood. Diabetes is a complex disease that is caused by several underlying factors, like obesity, lack of exercise, and family history amongst others. While high sugar intake is not a direct cause of diabetes, it can lead to obesity, which is one of the major risk factors for developing this condition. So, even if you never eat sweets, you can still get diabetes.

Myth:

- **Diabetes is a disease and like all diseases, it will go away.**

  - **Fact:** Diabetes is a lifelong disease that doesn't just go away. In the case of type 1 diabetes, your pancreas stops making insulin forever, therefore, those suffering from this type of diabetes will always need to take synthetic insulin. On the other hand, people with type 2 diabetes will always tend to have higher than normal blood sugar levels as their cells get resistant to insulin. However, type 2 diabetics can manage their blood sugar levels efficiently by changing unhealthy lifestyle habits, exercising regularly, eating healthy, fibrous food and monitoring their sugar levels frequently.

Myth:

- **I will never be able to eat rice and chapati again if I have diabetes.**

  - **Fact:** The ideal diet for diabetics is the same as everyone else - a well-balanced diet. This includes lots of veggies and fruits as well as eggs, lean meat, pulses, low-fat dairy items and fish. The most common Indian staples like chapati and rice can also be eaten by diabetics, however in moderation. Since both rice and chapati are rich in carbohydrates, they are believed to increase blood sugar levels, if consumed in excess amounts. Therefore, it's better to opt for brown rice rather than white rice as the latter is polished and processed. Also, chapatis made from chickpeas, corn, or barley are considered better than wheat.

Myth:

- **I am so young, I can't be diabetic.**

  - **Fact:** While it is widely believed that diabetes only strikes during old age, it's absolutely untrue. People of all ages can develop both type 1 and type 2 diabetes. Moreover, there has been an exponential rise in the cases of type 2 diabetes in children, teens, and young adults. In addition to this, the prevalence of type 1 diabetes is more in the younger population.

Myth:

- **Insulin cures diabetes!**

  - **Fact:** Diabetes is a chronic disease that has no cure. However, it can be managed to prevent any severe complications from arising. Insulin is a hormone that helps metabolise extra glucose out of your blood, where it can be used for energy. This helps in keeping the blood sugar levels under control.

With so many myths and rumours about diabetes flying around, it can be a little confusing for diabetics to figure out the best way to manage their condition. It's highly advisable to consult with your doctor before you commit to any lifestyle changes or treatment plans. For more information.

Some More Myths about Diabetes- Let's bust a myth.

Myth:

- **Diabetes is not serious.**

  - **Fact:** There is no such thing as "mild diabetes". All types of diabetes are serious and can lead to complications if not managed well. It can affect the quality of life and reduce life expectancy.

Myth:

- **All types of diabetes are the same.**

  - **Fact:** There are a number of types of diabetes. The most common are type 1, type 2 and gestational diabetes. Other forms of diabetes are less common. Each type of diabetes has different causes and may be managed in different ways. All types of diabetes are complex and serious, it needs management everyday.

Myth:

- **Pre-diabetes always leads to diabetes**

  - **Fact:** Pre-diabetes is a condition where blood sugar levels are higher than normal but not quite high enough to classify as diabetes. If left unchecked, pre-diabetes can develop into type 2 diabetes. Lifestyle changes can turn the tide. Regular physical activity and a more healthful diet can reverse pre-diabetes into the non diabetic stage very easily.

Myth:

- **I can't really have diabetes, I have no symptoms!**

  - **Fact:** Many people with diabetes have no symptoms. You can have diabetes for many years and not know it. Even if you do not have any symptoms, diabetes can cause damage to your body.

Myth:

- **I always know when my sugar is high or low, so I don't need to test it.**

  - **Fact:** You can't rely on how you're feeling when it comes to your blood sugar level. You may feel shaky, lightheaded, and dizzy because your blood sugar is low, or you may be coming down with a cold or the flu. You may urinate a lot because your glucose is high or because you have a bladder infection. The longer you have diabetes, the less accurate those feelings become. The only way to know for sure is to check your blood sugar.

Myth:

- **Losing weight means eating mostly salads.**

  - **Fact:** It's true that salad and vegetables are low calorie and can help with weight loss. But that alone will not help as you will feel hungry all that time and find it difficult to sustain it. Instead focus on a balanced diet that has more vegetables but also includes protein,fat and carbs.

Myth:

- **There are too many rules in a Diabetes diet.**

  - **Fact:** It is not that difficult to workout a diet plan. It is mainly about keeping your blood sugar levels as close to normal as possible. You may need to make adjustments to what you eat however, the new way of eating may not need that many changes. Just bare in mind to choose the foods that work well with your activities and any medications that you take.

Myth:

- **Fancy/fad diets leads to weight loss.**

  - **Fact:** There's no quick fix when it comes to health. Fad diets are not sustainable and provides only minor nutrients to the body and eliminates major nutrients which are necessary other metabolic functions.

Myth:

- **Eating breakfast is necessary to lose weight.**

  - **Fact:** Studies show that breakfast skippers tend to weigh more than breakfast eaters. It's also a myth that breakfast boosts metabolism and that eating multiple small meals makes you burn more calories throughout the day.

Myth:

- **Being on insulin means you don't have to make any lifestyle changes.**

    - **Fact:** When you are first diagnosed, your blood sugar may be controlled adequately by diet, exercise and oral medications. Eventually, however, your medications may not be as effective as they were, and you"ll likely need insulin injections to help control your blood sugar levels. Managing your diet and exercise with insulin is very important to help keep blood sugar levels in their target range and to help avoid complications.

Myth

- **Obesity cannot be reversed.**

    - **Fact:** While obesity is a chronic condition that requires lifelong management, it can be reversed with appropriate lifestyle changes. Sustainable weight loss is achievable through healthy eating habits and regular workout sessions.

Myth:

- **Weight loss supplements and pills are safe and effective.**

    - **Fact:** Weight loss supplements and pills are often marketed as quick fixes for obesity. However, most of these products lack scientific evidence to support their claims. The weight loss industry is largely unregulated; many supplements may contain potentially harmful ingredients or have unknown side effects.

Myth:

- **People with obesity are unhealthy and thin people are healthy.**

  - **Fact:** It's true that obesity increases your risk of several chronic illnesses, including type 2 diabetes, heart disease, and some cancers. However, plenty of people with obesity are metabolically healthy and plenty of thin people have these same chronic diseases.

Myth:

- **Fats don't matter**

  - **Fact:** According to the American Heart AssociationTrusted Source, having type 2 diabetes increases your risk of heart attack and stroke. Part of this link is due to the fact that many people with diabetes are also living with extra weight and often have high blood pressure or high cholesterol levels.

Myth:

- **Fruits are bad for diabetics.**

  - **Fact:** There are no as such forbidden fruits on a diabetes-friendly eating plan. However, it's true that some fruits contain more natural sugars hence have a high glycemic load than others, so you can enjoy them once in a while if you stick to the proper portion sizes and by having low glycemic load fruits and nuts along with it.

Myth:

- **Lifting weights is not a good way to improve your health or lose weight because it will make you "bulk up."**

  - **Fact:** Lifting weights or doing other activities 2 or 3 days a week that may help you build strong muscles, such as push-ups and some types of yoga, will not bulk you up. Only intense strength training, along with certain genes, can build large muscles. Like other kinds of physical activity, muscle-strengthening activities will help improve your health and also may help you control your weight by increasing the amount of energy-burning muscle.

Myth:

- **Diabetes is not serious**

  - **Fact:** There is no such thing as "mild diabetes". All types of diabetes are serious and can lead to complications if not managed well. It can affect the quality of life and reduce life expectancy.

Myth:

- **Artificial sweeteners are a healthier alternative to sugar.**

  - **Fact:** Artificial sweeteners should be consumed in moderation, as excessive use may have negative health effects and still impact blood sugar levels.

Myth:

- **Some types of diabetes are mild**

- **Fact**: There is no such thing as "mild diabetes". All types of diabetes are serious and can lead to complications if not managed well. It can affect the quality of life and reduce life expectancy.

Myth:

- **You will know if you have diabetes by your symptoms.**

  - **Fact**: Not true always. Type 2 diabetes often goes undiagnosed because it usually has few or no symptoms when it first develops.

Myth:

- **Only people with type 1 diabetes need insulin**

  - **Fact**: People who are suffering from type 1 diabetes depend on insulin replacements. They need to check their blood glucose levels several times during the day. On the other hand, type 2 is a progressive condition. 50% people with type 2 diabetes will need insulin 6-10 years of being diagnosed with diabetes because the pancreas produces less insulin over a period of time.

Myth:

- **Only older adults can get diabetes.**

  - **Fact**: While type 2 diabetes is more common in older adults, it's increasingly being diagnosed in younger people, including children and adolescents, due to rising obesity rates and sedentary lifestyle.

Myth:

- **People with diabetes can't eat carbohydrates.**

  - **Fact:** Carbohydrates can be included in a diabetic's diet, but portion control and choosing complex carbohydrates with fiber are important. Monitoring carbohydrate intake and managing blood sugar.

Myth:

- **People with diabetes cannot be active**

  - **Fact:** Once again, this is untrue. In fact, exercise is an important component in the management of diabetes. Among other things, exercise helps drive weight loss and reduces blood pressure, both of which are risk factors for complications. It can also help the body use insulin better.

Myth:

- **You can eat as much as you want if you exercise enough to manage diabetes.**

  - **Fact:** Exercise is important, but it's not a free pass to eat anything in unlimited quantities. Portion controlling and exercise together contribute to a balanced approach to diabetes management.

Myth:

- **Carbs Are Enemy For Diabetes.**

- **Fact:** Carbohydrate are essential part of a balanced diet.The type and quantity carb consumed matter more than simply their presence in Your diet. Whole grains can be beneficial in managing Diabetes.

APPENDIX

Basic Diabetic Diet regime

6:30 AM

1 tsp Methi seeds + 200 ml water + 1/2 tsp of cinnamon podwer.

(Soak it overnight and have it in the morning).

7:00 AM

1 cup (green tea) 300 ml.

3tsp fresubbin dm + 200 ml water.

+ (2) Marrie Biscuits Or (2) cream crackers Or (2) digestive biscuits.

Or (2) Nutrichoice 5 grains (Ragi nachni biscuits is fine) no Maida biscuits Or 2 methi khakhara.

9:30 AM

(2) egg white +1 vati Fenugreek leaves Or 2 brown bread slice OR 1 Chapatti.

(Or)

1 big bowl baggrys oats.

2 tsp oats + 3oo ml water + 2 almond + 1 walnut + 2 tsp skimmed milk powder + 6-8 black raisins + 1 tsp nachni Powder.

(Or) 1 Bowl bataka Poha (Or) 1 Bowl Upma. (Or) 2 Idli + 1 vati Sambhar (Or) 1 bowl cornflakes.

11:30 Am

Any 1 fruit (Avoid chickoo / custard apple / banana / mango / grapes / pineapple / Jack fruit, custard apple).

Include sweet lime / orange / watermelon / muskmelon / guava / apple / peach / plump / pear / papaya).

(Or)

1 glass Butter Milk.

12 :30 PM

2 1/2 tsp Fybogel + 200 Ml water + a pinch of methi seed powder.

1:00 PM

2 chapatti Or 1 Vat Rice Or 1 vati daliya khichadi.

+ 1 vati Saji.

+ 1 bowl salad.

+ 1 vati Dal(you can include lentil dal in your diet) Or 1 pcs chicken (Or) 1 pcs fish(grilled or roasted) (Or) 1 vati curd.

4 :00 PM

1 cup(green tea) 300 ml.

+ (2) Marrie Biscuits Or (2) cream crackers Or (2) digestive biscuits Or (2) Nutrichoice 5 grains (Ragi nachni biscuits is fine) no Maida biscuits.

6:00 PM

1 glass buttermilk

(3) tsp curd + 300 ml water (without salt).

Or 1 Vegetable Sandwich witch cheese (Brown Bread).

Or 1 bowl sprouted salads.

Or 1 Big Bowl vegetable soup.

Or 1 bowl Boil Corn.

Or 1 cheese toast sandwich (once in a week).

8:00 PM

2 1/2 tsp fybogel + 200 ml water + a pinch of methi seed powder.

8:30 PM

2 chapatti (or) 2 Brown Bread slice (Or) 1 Bowl daliya khichadi (OR) 1 Bowl biryani.

+ 1 bowl sabji.

+ 1 bowl dal (Or) 1 pcs chicken (Or) 1 pcs fish (grilled or roasted).

+ 1 vati salad.

11 :00 PM

100ml milk + 200 ml water + 2 almonds +3 walnuts +5 TO 6 black raisins + 2 tsp sabja.

Some Important Suggestions

Few common sense HEALTH TIPS FOR All

A. Two things to check often:
(1) Your blood pressure
(2) Your blood sugar

B. Three things reduced to minimum:
(1) salt
(2) sugar
(3) starch (Carbohydrates)

C. Four things to increase:
(1) Greens
(2) Veggies
(3) fruits
(4) Nuts

D. Three things to forget:
(1) Your age
(2) your past
(3) your grudges

E. Three things to have:
(1) True Friends
(2) Loving family
(3) Positive thoughts

F. Four acts to stay healthy:
(1) Fasting
(2) Laughing
(3) Exercise
(4) Weight loss

G. Four things not to wait for:
(1) Don't wait till you are sleepy to sleep
(2) Don't wait till you are tired to rest
(3) Don't wait till your friend is sick to go to see him.
(4) Don't wait for problems to pray to God.

TAKE CARE OF YOURSELF.. & STAY YOUNG!!

Further Suggestions

- Eat regular meals to keep your blood glucose and metabolism on track.

- Prefer brown rice to traditional white rice. An increase in fiber content will improve glycemic control.

- Include variety of whole grains like oats, cracked wheat, barley, millets like ragi etc in meals.

- Make your chapati nutritious by using multigrain atta.

- While consuming starchy vegetables like potatoes, peas, corn etc remember to count them as carbohydrates and cut down on rice eaten in the same meal. Consider the portions:

  - One serving (1 cup cooked or 1 cup raw veggies) of non-starchy vegetables includes green leafy vegetables, lady fingers, cabbage, cauliflower, brinjal, peppers, tomato, bottle gourd and family etc.

  - One serving (1/2 cup cooked) of starchy vegetables includes corn, peas, potato, sweet potato, yam, beetroot, beans.

- Practice oil rotation as complete dependence on just one oil does not ensure optimal intake of fatty acids. Use oil choosing one from each group:

  - A: Sunflower/ Safflower/ Corn oil/ Rice Bran

  - B: Mustard/ Groundnut/ Olive/ Canola

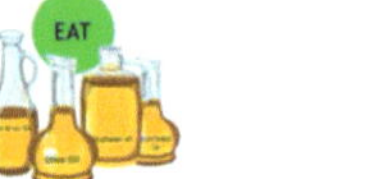

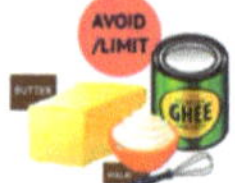

- Avoid deep frying, use saute, grilling, roasting, steaming or pressure cooking as cooking methods.

- Include proteins from lean meats, skinless poultry, sea food, egg whites, sprouted pulses, soya products, unsalted nuts & low fat dairy.

- Choose fresh fruits over juices.

- Maintain a log of meals and blood glucose levels to understand your fluctuations better.

- Carbohydrates in food is a main contributor to rise in blood glucose after eating, it is advisable to distribute carbohydrate intake throughout the day & avoid one big heavy meal.

- When eating out, prefer smaller portions to larger ones. Plan your meals in advance to avoid carbohydrate and fat overload.

- Avoid aerated and high calorie drinks and choose healthier options like soups, buttermilk, coconut water & fresh lime.

- Flaxseeds and Chia seeds are loaded with healthy fats, fiber, protein and essential minerals. Add them to smoothies, milkshakes, buttermilk, yogurt.

- Watch out for symptoms of hypoglycemia! If blood sugar drops below 70mg/dl(hypoglycemia) treat yourself with 3 teaspoons of sugar/honey or 1 cup fruit juice or regular soft drink.

- If planning to consume sweets, replace yogurt with dessert sweetened with artificial sweetener and keep the portion sizes small.